The Uncomplicated Guide to Diabetes Complications

△.American Diabetes Association.
Cure • Care • Commitment™

Director, Book Publishing, John Fedor; *Associate Director, Consumer Books,* Sherrye Landrum; *Editor,* Sherrye Landrum; *Production Manager,* Peggy M. Rote; *Composition,* Circle Graphics, Inc.; *Cover Design,* Kathy Tresnak; *Printer,* Transcontinental Printing

Printed in Canada

1 3 5 7 9 10 8 6 4 2

The suggestions and information contained in this publication are generally consistent with the *Clinical Practice Recommendations* and other policies of the American Diabetes Association, but they do not represent the policy or position of the Association or any of its boards or committees. Reasonable steps have been taken to ensure the accuracy of the information presented. However, the American Diabetes Association cannot ensure the safety or efficacy of any product or service described in this publication. Individuals are advised to consult a physician or other appropriate health care professional before undertaking any diet or exercise program or taking any medication referred to in this publication. Professionals must use and apply their own professional judgment, experience, and training and should not rely solely on the information contained in this publication before prescribing any diet, exercise, or medication. The American Diabetes Association—its officers, directors, employees, volunteers, and members—assumes no responsibility or liability for personal or other injury, loss, or damage that may result from the suggestions or information in this publication.

♾ The paper in this publication meets the requirements of the ANSI Standard Z39.48-1992 (permanence of paper).

ADA titles may be purchased for business or promotional use or for special sales. To purchase this book in large quantities, or for custom editions of this book with your logo, contact Lee Romano Sequeira, Special Sales & Promotions, at the address below, or at LRomano@diabetes.org or 703-299-2046.

American Diabetes Association
1701 North Beauregard Street
Alexandria, Virginia 22311

Library of Congress Cataloging-in-Publication Data

The uncomplicated guide to diabetes complications / edited by Marvin E. Levin and Michael A. Pfeifer. —2nd ed.
    p. cm.
  Includes index.
  ISBN 1-58040-133-3 (pbk. : alk. paper)
    1. Diabetes—Complications—Popular works. I. Levin, Marvin E., 1924- II. Pfeifer, Michael A.

  RC660.4 .U53 2002
  616.4'62—dc21   2002074397

Contents

Introduction

Two miracles, the discoveries of insulin and antibiotics, have significantly prolonged the life of people with diabetes. That is good news. The bad news is that longer life spans allow many people with diabetes to develop complications of the disease.

But there's more good news: Diabetic complications can be prevented, and they can be treated. This requires you to be better educated about your risks and what you can do to lower them. It also requires the expertise of many medical specialties, so to help you, we have gathered in this book the knowledge and contributions of many world-renowned specialists.

The complications that commonly occur in diabetes include eye disease, now the leading cause of blindness in the U.S.; atherosclerosis, hardening of the arteries, which can lead to heart attack and stroke; loss of nerve function, particularly in the lower extremities, which can lead to painless injury, ulcers, infection, gangrene, and amputation; and kidney disease, now the leading reason for dialysis. Diabetes puts you at much greater risk of developing heart disease and poor circulation. Every step you take each day to control your blood glucose and blood pressure levels improves your overall health for the present and the future.

We want to help you prevent the complications of diabetes. In addition to improved quality of life, this would result in saving billions of dollars a year in Medicare costs. What you need is good blood glucose control and to catch complications early by checking the following regularly:

1. A1C (glycated hemoglobin)
2. Blood pressure
3. LDL cholesterol
4. Dilated eye examination
5. Urinary protein
6. Monofilament testing

To further improve your chances of not having a complication, stop smoking and get patient education about living with diabetes (including meal planning). Don't wait until symptoms occur. Any of the six tests above can give abnormal results before you have any symptoms. The key to success is to catch it early. That is the time to treat the complication.

This book deals with how to prevent complications and, if problems occur, how they can and should be treated. It also points out many of the things your doctor and other health care providers should be doing to help you and to treat complications. All of these treatments should be discussed with and prescribed by your doctors. Never use them without medical supervision or assistance.

As you read the book, you will see that the bottom line—and there is always a bottom line—is repeated over and over: **The most important thing you can do to help prevent complications is to achieve good blood glucose control. It's the best way to manage them, too.**

List of Contributors

Lloyd Paul Aiello, MD, PhD
Paul D. Baker
Jeffrey L. Barnett, MD
Jose Biller, MD, FACP
Michael Camilleri, MD
Culley C. Carson, MD
Jerry D. Cavallerano, OD, PhD
Samuel Dagogo-Jack, MD, FACP
Eva L. Feldman, MD, PhD
Karen Flavin, RN, CCRC
Eli A. Friedman, MD
Robert G. Frykberg, DPM, MPH
Martha M. Funnel, MS, RN, CDE
Edward M. Geltman, MD
Saul M. Genuth, MD
Gary W. Gibbons, MD
M. Gilbert Grand, MD
Douglas A. Greene, MD
Charlotte Hayes, MMSc, MS, RD, CDE
Joan M. Heins, MA, RD, CDE
Irl B. Hirsch, MD
Mami A. Iwamoto, MD
Sheilah A. Janus
Erick Janisse, CPed, BOCO
Lois Jovanovic, MD

Jeffrey A. Levin, DMD
Benjamin A. Lipsky, MD
Betsy B. Love, MD
Dordaneh Maleki, MD
Mark E. Molitch, MD
Michael J. Mueller, PT, PhD
Edward R. Newton, MD
Mark Peyrot, PhD
Laurinda M. Poirier, RN, MPH, CDE
Venkatraman Rajkumar, MD
Richard R. Rubin, PhD, CDE
Lee J. Sanders, DPM
Leslie R. Schover, PhD
Patricia Schreiner-Engel, PhD
R. Gary Sibbald, MD
David R. Sinacore, PT, PhD
James R. Sowers, MD
Ilana P. Spector, PhD
Mark A. Sperling, MD
Martin J. Stevens, MD
David E.R. Sutherland, MD, PhD
Aruna Venkatesh, MD
Aaron Vinik, MD, PhD, FCP, FACP
Katherine V. Williams, MD
Rena R. Wing, PhD

1

Acute Complications: DKA and HHS

Case study

MJ is 47 years old and has had type 1 diabetes for 20 years. She is suffering from an intestinal flu with vomiting and hasn't eaten in 24 hours. Because she hasn't eaten, she has mistakenly decided not to take any insulin. Now she feels really awful, dizzy, and short of breath. The vomiting continues. She calls her health care provider, who suspects diabetic ketoacidosis (DKA) and tells her to go to the emergency room immediately.

Case study

LP is 72 years old, lives alone, and was just diagnosed with type 2 diabetes last week. He has been taking prednisone, a steroid, for 4 weeks for another serious condition. Now he is extremely thirsty and urinating often. He feels exhausted. Sensing that something is wrong, he goes to see his physician who finds that his blood pressure is low and his blood glucose level is 925 mg/dl. By now he is sleepy and lethargic. He is experiencing a hyperosmolar hyperglycemic state (HHS).

What is DKA?

DKA occurs when blood glucose levels rise too high and the body becomes very dehydrated and begins to burn excessive amounts of fat for energy. This causes the body to produce ketones, acid products of burning fat. The large excess of ketones and acids give this condition the name ketoacidosis. When severe, this can be life-threatening.

What causes DKA?

When you don't have enough insulin or it's not working right, glucose cannot get from your bloodstream into the cells. The cells send out a distress signal. Replacement glucose is made in the liver and flows into the blood. In DKA, both factors—slower exit of glucose from the blood and faster entrance of glucose from the liver—raise glucose levels in the blood. Exactly how high they can go depends on still another organ, the kidney.

The role of the kidney is complicated to explain (Figure 1-1). The kidney saves glucose, because the glucose molecule is essential to so many body functions. Normally, glucose is filtered out of the blood in one part of the kidney and returned to the blood in another part. However, when blood glucose (BG) levels rise above 180 mg/dl, the kidney cannot reclaim it all and lets the excess glucose go in the urine. This is how the kidney helps keep BG from going even higher than it already has.

The glucose must be dissolved in water to be excreted. So, your body needs more water. The glucose excreted in urine takes with it huge amounts of water and sodium chloride (salt). Sodium chloride keeps enough water in the bloodstream so that the blood pumped by the heart can carry sufficient oxygen and nutrients to every cell in the body. As more and more water and sodium chloride are lost in the urine, you become dried out (dehydrated), limiting further what the kidney can do. That is why two of the symptoms of uncontrolled diabetes are extreme

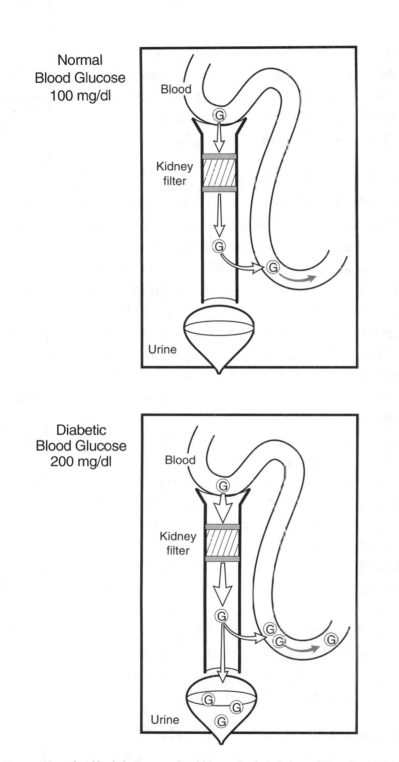

Normal
Blood Glucose
100 mg/dl

Blood

Kidney
filter

Urine

Diabetic
Blood Glucose
200 mg/dl

Blood

Kidney
filter

Urine

Figure 1-1. When blood glucose goes above a certain level, the kidney releases glucose in the urine.

thirst and excessive urination. Finally, in DKA, the kidney excretes more fluid than you drink, and your body becomes severely dehydrated. The kidney cannot filter enough glucose out of the blood. Your BG can rise to levels of 400–1,000 mg/dl (and, although rarely, sometimes higher).

What does ketoacidosis mean?

Ordinarily, the body burns fat and carbohydrates to get carbon dioxide and water. To keep this process going efficiently, some glucose must be added to the fuel mix, which requires insulin. When insulin either is unavailable or doesn't work properly, two things happen. First, fat is released from storage cells and broken down for use as an energy source. But, there's too much fat, and the liver can't burn it completely. The process stops at a chemical half-way point—becoming ketoacids—before carbon dioxide and water are formed (Figure 1-2). The ketoacids are made in huge quantities, and they pile up in the blood after they are released from the liver. The ketoacids are the *keto* in ketoacidosis. They also are excreted in your urine and can be detected by a urine ketone test.

Now, what about *acidosis*? The two ketoacids are relatively strong acids. Think of them like acetic acid in vinegar. The body cannot tolerate ketoacids for long. They must be neutralized, and the body converts them to carbon dioxide, which is exhaled by the lungs. People with DKA must breathe more rapidly and deeply to get rid of the extra carbon dioxide. Acetone is also exhaled. This causes the breath to have a fruity odor. If the lungs did not get rid of the extra carbon dioxide, the high acid level of the blood would poison all the body cells, and life would cease. That's why insulin was truly a magical life-saving drug in the first few years of its use—and it still is.

What puts you at risk for developing DKA?

Not having enough insulin puts you at risk for DKA. Most cases occur in people with type 1 diabetes. In some instances,

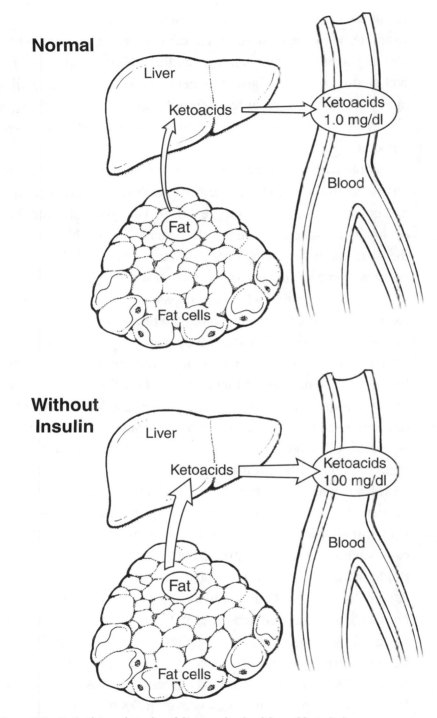

Normal

Liver

Ketoacids → Ketoacids 1.0 mg/dl

Blood

Fat

Fat cells

Without Insulin

Liver

Ketoacids → Ketoacids 100 mg/dl

Blood

Fat

Fat cells

Figure 1-2. Ketoacids are a byproduct of the incomplete breakdown of fat in the liver.

the individuals did not even know they had diabetes—for example, school-age children sent off to camp, where neither they nor their counselors recognized that frequent urination or bed-wetting could be signs of diabetes. Most people with undiagnosed diabetes have suffered from frequent urination, thirst, loss of weight, and blurred vision for 4–8 weeks before they see a doctor.

People with type 1 diabetes who have an interruption in their insulin treatment get DKA. The time between stopping insulin and going into DKA varies a great deal. The quickest example occurs in insulin pump patients. If the catheter gets blocked or the pump stops delivering insulin for any reason, DKA can occur within 6–12 hours, because the insulin used in the pump is rapid-acting insulin, which disappears rapidly from the body. (Note: This is not a reason to avoid the insulin pump, just be aware.) In contrast, DKA may take several days to develop after stopping NPH, lente, ultralente insulin, or insulin glargine because they hang around longer in the skin. The more years a person has had type 1 diabetes, the quicker DKA is likely to develop when treatment is interrupted, because there are no beta cells left to provide even the small amount of insulin it takes to prevent ketoacidosis.

Even if you take all prescribed insulin doses, DKA can still happen. This is usually brought about by an illness—such as strep throat or intestinal flu. Flu is especially bad because it causes vomiting and/or diarrhea, both of which decrease body fluids and make dehydration worse. The stress of an illness or surgery causes your body to release stress hormones, including cortisone, glucagon, epinephrine, and growth hormone. Each of these opposes insulin action. Together, they raise BG and ketoacid levels. In type 1 patients who have little or no insulin reserve, DKA can develop quickly unless extra insulin is given. Patients with type 2 diabetes can develop DKA even though their bodies make insulin. They have insulin resistance; their bodies are resistant to the action of insulin, and need additional insulin to correct the elevated BG and DKA.

As in the first case study, people cause DKA by not taking insulin when they are vomiting or have diarrhea. They make the mistake of thinking that because they are not eating, their blood glucose will be low. If you don't inject insulin, your BG will rise even if you haven't eaten.

On rare occasions, no illness can be found, but DKA still occurs. The stress causing DKA may be emotional, such as a distressing school, work, or family situation. Emotional upsets can cause repeated episodes of DKA weeks or months apart, and your physician or family may need to help you unveil the problem to yourself. You may need professional help.

DKA is more likely to occur in adolescents, who are trying to deal with the physical, psychological, and social changes of puberty in addition to diabetes. The problem is especially dangerous when it leads teenagers to stop taking insulin as a means of testing themselves, their diabetes, and their family's love and attention. Teenage girls will sometimes allow themselves to have higher-than-normal glucose levels, so they can eat whatever they want and not gain weight. The problem is that it takes very little to send them into ketoacidosis. They are seen multiple times a year in the emergency room in DKA. If the parents or doctor recognize what is happening they can help the young person balance their responsibilities better.

Can people with type 2 diabetes develop DKA?

Yes, DKA can occur in older people with type 2 diabetes. It is usually brought on by major medical illness such as a heart attack, trauma such as a hip fracture, or an emergency surgery such as appendicitis. When there is no obvious cause for DKA, your physician must look for unusual infections that may be masked by the DKA itself. These include meningitis, serious external ear infections, fungal infections in the nose, dental infections, and even rectal abscesses. Finally, adrenal or pituitary glands may secrete excess amounts of the stress hormones mentioned above. In rare cases, this may present as DKA. You might say that while DKA itself is easy to recognize, identifying its cause may take detective work by you and your diabetes care team.

What are the symptoms of DKA?

With few exceptions, you feel awful. Rising BG levels have caused frequent urination and extreme thirst. Dehydration causes a parched tongue, weakness, and dizziness on standing. The high blood-acid level causes nausea, vomiting, and, rarely, abdominal pain so severe that it mimics diseases such as appendicitis. Diarrhea is not a symptom of DKA, and its presence may point to gastroenteritis as the illness causing DKA. You hyperventilate to "blow off" the carbon dioxide being formed from neutralizing the acid in the blood. This often gives you the sensation of being short of breath. After many hours of high BG, the brain cells also become dehydrated and function abnormally. Lethargy, sleepiness, and confusion result and can end up as coma. Someone must get you to a hospital immediately.

How is DKA treated?

The most pressing need is for intravenous water and salt. This is given rapidly in the first 1–2 hours of treatment to restore circulation to all body tissues. This improves blood flow to the kidneys so they can remove glucose from the blood more efficiently (Figure 1-1). More intravenous fluid is given slowly over 8–24 hours until all the body water losses have been made up. This may require as much as 5–10 quarts of fluid.

Next you need insulin. This is also given intravenously whenever possible to guarantee a quick and reliable effect. Besides bringing BG down to a reasonable range (150–250 mg/dl), the insulin stops the release and the burning of so much fat. In turn, this stops production of ketoacids and gradually corrects the acidosis. It is important to get potassium, too. Otherwise, potassium levels may fall to dangerously low levels in the blood because the cells soak it up so quickly. A very low blood potassium level can interfere with the action of the heart. Occasionally, phosphate is given. The rarest are circumstances where magnesium falls to critically low levels in the blood and causes heart irregularities that require emergency treatment with intravenous magnesium.

The acidosis is gradually corrected by insulin treatment. Occasionally, however, the level of acid is so high that it is endangering you. A sterile liquid form of baking soda may be given intravenously to neutralize the excess of acid and allow time for insulin to work. This is not recommended for young children, however.

Your pulse, blood pressure, and mental status are checked hourly. Blood samples to check glucose, acid levels, potassium, and phosphate are taken regularly. To prevent vomiting, no fluids are allowed by mouth. All intravenous fluids given and all urine passed must be measured and charted to be sure that you are regaining body fluids. Electrocardiograms (ECGs) are performed. It is small wonder that most patients get very little rest and are often very tired and somewhat cranky the next day.

How can you prevent DKA?

Learn when to be concerned about DKA and how to check for it. Ask your physician to help you make a sick-day plan. Any illness, even the common cold, should trigger you and your family's early warning system. Fever, nausea, and vomiting even one time are danger flags. If you have any of these symptoms, check BG and urine ketones immediately. If BG level is less than 250 mg/dl and urine ketones are negative, take your usual insulin doses and continue to monitor BG and urine ketones every 4 hours until the illness has passed. Drink fluids of all kinds in generous amounts. If you vomit a second time, your BG increases to more than 250 mg/dl, or the urine test for ketones becomes positive, call your health care provider at once for advice.

You must pay attention to vomiting, because it increases your risk of dehydration. Diarrhea may add to the loss of fluids and salts. Infants and young children are particularly vulnerable to DKA because they normally begin with less fluid in their bodies. Also, elderly people have less kidney function to start with. You can replace lost water and salt with bouillon (one cube in 8 oz water). Gatorade or similar products or a solution of glucose, salt, baking soda, and potassium recommended by the World Health Organization usually works well. Small amounts of fluid taken frequently, for example, 3 ounces every 20–30 minutes for an adult, are better for you than large amounts drunk rapidly. If BG is below normal, drink high carbohydrate fluids, such as fruit juices, regular sodas, or tea with sugar, alternating with fluids that contain salt, such as bouillon.

Some physicians provide you with prescriptions in advance for medications for nausea and vomiting such as rectal suppositories and instructions on how to use them. Stopping the vomiting helps prevent DKA because it reduces the risk of dehydration.

The other rule is: Never stop your insulin injections because of loss of appetite, nausea, vomiting, or fear of hypoglycemia. You may need to change your insulin dose. That is why you need to check your BG and urine ketones often to navigate through this dangerous period, especially if you have signs of DKA. You may need to check every 2 hours even in the middle of the night, and call in the results to your health care team. They should give you instructions about doses of insulin to take and instructions for future doses, depending on later BG and urine ketone test results.

When you call the doctor have up-to-the-minute BG and urine ketone results and an estimate of how much and what kind of fluids you have drunk. If you all work together as a true team, the risk of DKA can be minimized or eliminated. If the infection is bacterial, for example strep throat, antibiotics may speed your recovery, so get prescriptions filled immediately. Once your BG has been in a safe range (100–200 mg/dl) for a few hours and no ketones are in your urine, the danger of DKA is generally over.

What are the signs that DKA is getting worse?

Continued vomiting, complaints of shortness of breath, and excessive sleepiness. Your doctor may note breathlessness and a dulling of mental processes by listening to you on the telephone. That's why he should talk with you and not a family member. If these symptoms appear, you need to go to the emergency room for help.

What is hyperosmolar hyperglycemic state (HHS)?

Many of the things already said about DKA apply to HHS. The first H stands for *hyperosmolar* and is a technical way of saying that all of the chemicals contained in blood are now dissolved in much less water. Because of this, water is drawn into the blood from the body cells so that the patient is very dehydrated. The blood may become so thick that it clots easily, which can cause strokes and heart attacks.

Hyperglycemic (the second H) means that BG levels are too high. HHS has a higher average blood glucose (900 mg/dl or higher) than DKA. BG can go higher for several reasons. HHS develops more slowly and gradually. The thirsty patient seems to prefer sweet liquids with higher carbohydrate content. The function of the kidneys is more greatly reduced because the patient becomes more dehydrated. And the patient or caregivers ignore or mistake the symptoms for something else and wait too long to see the health care team. By the time they do, the loss of salt and especially of plain water from the body can be enormous.

Ketoacids are not produced in HHS and do not build up in the blood. The reason may be that these patients have type 2 diabetes. They still make a small amount of insulin. The lack of high acid levels in the blood is a reason for the long delay in getting care: you are not alerted by nausea and vomiting that something is very wrong. HHS more often leads to *coma* (a state of unconsciousness) than does DKA. It is more life threatening and harder to reverse.

Who is at risk of developing HHS?

The typical patient is an elderly person, who is often living alone or in a nursing home and may be unaware that she even has type 2 diabetes. A heart attack or an infection that has spread into the bloodstream from a site such as the urinary tract or a foot ulcer may start the process. Certain drugs can contribute to a steep rise in BG, too. Examples are prednisone or other steroids, diuretics such as hydrochlorothiazide, and anticonvulsant medication such as dilantin.

What are the symptoms of HHS?

You are usually more dehydrated—literally dried out—with prunelike wrinkled skin. You are more likely to be in shock; that is, to have very low blood pressure with poor blood flow to many organs. Coma is much more frequent. The brain may be so affected by the dehydration that seizures, paralysis, and other neurological problems can occur. Many patients seem to have had a stroke; yet with complete treatment, the abnormal neurological signs can disappear completely. It may take several days. HHS is a more serious acute complication of diabetes than is DKA, and the chances of recovering from it are not as good, even with correct treatment.

What is the treatment for HHS?

Usually only small amounts of insulin are required. HHS patients need emergency fluid flowing to their tissues to get them out of shock and to restore normal blood flow to the heart, brain, kidneys, liver, and limbs. Because elderly patients with type 2 diabetes usually have atherosclerosis, improving blood flow and oxygen delivery quickly is vital to prevent complete blockage of one of these narrowed major arteries. A blockage can cause a heart attack, stroke, or kidney failure.

How can you prevent HHS?

You, your family, nursing home personnel, and health care professionals all need to be educated about this condition. Elderly people should be tested for diabetes periodically. Paying close attention to the welfare of elderly relatives who have diabetes can prevent many cases. Aides and nurses in facilities that care for the aged must be alert to frequent urination or the abrupt appearance of incontinence. Elderly people do not experience thirst as well as younger people do when the body needs water. They and their caregivers need to note how much fluid they drink. Don't write off a decline in mental status as "senile dementia" without checking for high BG. Likewise, don't dismiss a complaint of dizziness, especially on standing, which could signal a low volume of blood. We need to be as concerned that a person is having a "glucose attack" as we are for heart attacks and the recently coined term *brain attacks*. Nothing is easier or more certain to help a patient than bringing down a dangerously high blood glucose level—provided treatment is started in time.

What is lactic acidosis (LA)?

Lactic acidosis is a condition like DKA. Lactic acid is normally present in blood and muscle tissue as a byproduct of the metabolism of glucose. When some event such as a heart attack limits oxygen to the blood and tissues, lactic acid levels can build up. LA occurring with diabetes is rare. The symptoms can be like those of DKA. The high blood acid level causes nausea and vomiting, and the patient has to breathe hard to get rid of the carbon dioxide being released.

Who is at risk for developing LA?

Rarely, LA will appear in people with type 2 diabetes who take metformin, a diabetes pill. Metformin (Glucophage) is an effective and safe medication for people with type 2 diabetes. If the kidney is not functioning, however, problems can arise. For example, JD is taking metformin for his type 2 diabetes. He also has vascular disease and had dye-contrast X rays taken yesterday. Today the dye is causing kidney problems. Because he was not told to stop the metformin before the test, he develops LA.

Although LA is a very uncommon complication of taking metformin, it does happen. **You should not be taking metformin if you have kidney disease, liver disease, alcoholism, cardiovascular disease, or if you are pregnant.**

What are the symptoms of LA?

The symptoms of LA are nausea, vomiting, abdominal pain, and lethargy. The signs are shock, severe anemia, low blood pressure, and hyperventilation. LA can have serious effects on the heart and blood circulation, affecting heart rhythm, heart rate, and blood pressure.

What is the treatment for LA?

As with DKA, it is important to restore fluid for circulation to provide oxygen and nutrients to all body tissues. Salt and water may be given intravenously along with a sterile form of baking soda to neutralize the acid. Using a dialysis machine to cleanse the blood of metformin and lactic acid is sometimes an effective treatment.

This chapter was written by Saul M. Genuth, MD.

2

Hypoglycemia

How does your body avoid BG going too low?

When you eat, the rise in glucose tells the pancreas to release insulin (a hormone) into the blood. Insulin, natural or injected, opens the door to the cells and lowers the amount of glucose in the blood. There are several other hormones—*glucagon, epinephrine, cortisol,* and *growth hormone*—that work to raise glucose levels (Table 2-1). These hormones are released into the blood when BG gets too low. They are called *counter-regulatory* or *stress hormones.*

Glucagon is made in the pancreas, as is insulin, but in a different type of cell. It raises glucose levels within a few minutes. *Epinephrine,* also known as adrenaline, is made by the adrenal glands. Epinephrine works within minutes. It stops insulin release and causes cells not to respond to insulin. When it is released to treat hypoglycemia, it causes rapid heartbeat, sweating, and a feeling of anxiety. *Cortisol* is released by another part of the adrenal glands and acts more slowly to raise BG. *Growth hormone* is released by the pituitary gland. It also acts more slowly to raise BG levels.

What are the symptoms of hypoglycemia?

Symptoms of hypoglycemia are usually divided into those that affect the body and those that affect the brain (Table 2-2).

Table 2-1. Hormones Controlling Glucose Levels

Lowers BG	Raises BG
Insulin	Glucagon
	Epinephrine (adrenaline)
	Cortisol
	Growth hormone

Among the bodily symptoms, rapid and forceful heartbeat, hunger, sweating, and nausea are the most common. Most of these symptoms are related to the release of epinephrine.

When the brain is affected, symptoms may range from light-headedness and anxiety to confusion, loss of consciousness, and even seizures. These symptoms occur when the brain doesn't get enough glucose. The bodily symptoms depend on how low the glucose levels go and how rapidly they are falling.

Table 2-2. Symptoms of Hypoglycemia

Bodily Symptoms	Central Nervous System Symptoms
Rapid heartbeat	Light-headedness
Sweating	Confusion
Tremors	Headache
Anxiety	Loss of consciousness (coma)
Hunger	Seizures
Nausea	Delayed reflexes
	Slurred speech

The Uncomplicated Guide to Diabetes Complications

What is hypoglycemia unawareness?

People who often have hypoglycemia may lose all symptoms, and the first sign is that they become confused. This is called *hypoglycemia unawareness* and can be dangerous. If you are driving a car or operating heavy machinery, even the slightest bit of confusion or delayed reaction may cause an accident.

Some people develop hypoglycemia unawareness **because** they have lots of hypoglycemic episodes. The body gradually adapts to hypoglycemia, so it takes lower and lower blood glucose to cause a release of epinephrine and warning symptoms. However, the brain does not adapt. The first symptom is confusion, making it more difficult for you to help yourself.

In people who have nerve damage (autonomic neuropathy), epinephrine is not released on time and there are no warning symptoms. Often glucagon is also not released, so the hypoglycemia may last longer (chapter 12).

If you have hypoglycemia unawareness, check your BG frequently and wear diabetes identification. Always check your BG before you drive and every 1–2 hours on long trips. You need to protect yourself and others.

Do people without diabetes develop hypoglycemia?

Even if someone fasts for 3 days, glucose levels don't fall to hypoglycemic levels. With prolonged starvation, glucose levels may dip below 50 mg/dl, but this rarely happens outside of countries plagued by malnutrition.

In some people, glucose may be absorbed too rapidly from the intestine, triggering a sharp rise in insulin. The large amount of insulin rapidly sends glucose into the cells, but no more glucose comes in from the intestine, and there is an imbalance. Low BG occurs. This low usually lasts a few minutes up to an hour or two because the counterregulatory hormones stimulate the liver to release more glucose into the blood. And, the low glucose level shuts off further insulin release. If you have this type of hypoglycemia, avoid eating a lot of carbohydrate at one meal, so you don't have a sharp rise in BG. Eating high fiber foods and small snacks between meals may help.

Do diabetes pills cause hypoglycemia?

Sulfonylureas and meglitinides can cause low blood sugar.

Sulfonylureas

Sulfonylureas stimulate the pancreas to release insulin (Table 2-3). They can cause hypoglycemia. This may occur 2–3 hours after a meal if the sulfonylurea causes the pancreas to release too much insulin. Don't skip a meal or take too much medication. This hypoglycemia is usually mild and is detected by symptoms or checking BG. Treat by reducing the dose of medication or eating a snack between meals. You may be given acarbose or miglitol to delay glucose absorption from

Table 2-3. Oral Medications Used to Treat Diabetes

Stimulates More Insulin	Insulin Sensitizers	Slows Glucose Absorption
Sulfonylureas	Biguanides	alpha-glucosidase inhibitors
Tolbutamide (Orinase)	Metformin (Glucophage)	Acarbose (Precose)
Chlorpropamide (Diabinase)	Thiazolidinediones	Miglitol (Glyset)
Tolazamide (Tolinase)	Rosiglitazone (Avandia)	
Glyburide (generic)	Pioglitazone (Actos)	
Glipizide (generic)		
Glipizide-GITS (Glucotrol XL)		
Glimepiride (Amaryl)		
Meglitinides		
Repaglinide (Prandin)		
Nateglinide (Starlex)		

the intestines, so there'll be a closer match between the timing of insulin and glucose.

People taking the longer-acting medications chlorpropamide and glyburide who have kidney failure or renal impairment can have hypoglycemia. Prolonged hypoglycemia occurs in older people who may skip meals, and it may last for many hours, or more than a day. Treatment is to eat carbohydrate immediately, but hospitalization may be necessary.

Two drugs that act like sulfonylureas and can cause hypoglycemia are repaglinide (Prandin) and nateglinide (Starlex). They act rapidly, so they must be taken with a meal.

Other oral agents—metformin, acarbose, miglitol, 'glitazones

People who take metformin (Glucophage), acarbose (Precose), rosiglitazone (Avandia) or pioglitazone (Actos) should not have hypoglycemia. However, if you take one of these pills with a sulfonylurea or with insulin, you can develop hypoglycemia. Anyone taking acarbose or miglitol must treat hypoglycemia with pure glucose tablets and not juice, candy, or table sugar.

What causes hypoglycemia in people taking insulin?

Hypoglycemia results from taking too much insulin, eating too little food, skipping a meal, or exercising more than you had planned.

Although the usual times of insulin action are listed in Table 2-4, these times vary from one person to another, making lows quite possible. You may find there is a variation depending on where you inject insulin—absorption is fastest from the abdomen and slowest from the buttocks—and whether there is any scar tissue at the site of injection. If you exercise within 30–60 minutes of the injection, blood flow to the legs and arms is increased, and the insulin may be more rapidly absorbed than you expect, causing low BG.

Table 2-4. Types of Insulin

Type	Onset (h)	Peak (h)	Duration (h)
Rapid acting			
lispro	5–30 min	1/2–2 1/2	3–4
aspart	5–15 min	1/2–1	1–3
Regular	1/2–1	2–3	3–6
NPH	2–4	4–10	10–16
Lente	2–4	4–12	12–18
Ultralente	6–10	10–16	18–20
Insulin Glargine	2–4	Peakless	24

How do you adjust insulin and food for exercise?

You'll need to keep records of BG levels and exercise so you and your doctor can see your patterns. Here's an example of what to do. A 16-year-old patient takes 12 units of NPH in the morning before breakfast and 8 units of NPH before supper. When he knows he has basketball practice after school, he lowers his morning dose of NPH by 4 units and his evening dose of NPH by 2 units. He also decreases his lunch rapid-acting insulin by 2 units and his supper rapid-acting insulin by 1 unit. He has learned that this helps prevent hypoglycemia during practice and later that evening. Exercise can lower glucose levels for up to 24 hours. He knows that, so he'll eat a bigger bedtime snack than usual. He also carries glucose tablets with him in case his game is more vigorous or longer than expected.

How do you treat hypoglycemia?

When you have symptoms or get a low BG reading, eat 15–20 grams of carbohydrate right away. Wait for 15–20 minutes. Check your BG level then to be sure it has risen enough. If it hasn't, eat another 15–20 grams of carbohydrate.

Can you prevent going too low when driving?

Check your BG before driving and every 2 hours on long trips. Always have something to eat where you can reach it in the car. By the time you feel low, your nervous system reaction times are decreased and your ability to respond quickly is not good.

Pull off the road. Get in the passenger seat, eat, check your BG, and wait at least 20–30 minutes until you are feeling normal before driving again. The last thing to do when you feel low is to decide that you are almost home or to the restaurant or store, and drive the rest of the way. That is a sure way to have an accident.

What can others do to help with hypoglycemia?

The rule for helpers is: **Never force juice or food into the mouth of an unconscious person.** If you are unconscious or unable to eat, you need an injection of glucagon. Ask your doctor to prescribe it and teach friends or family members how to give it. If you do not respond, they should call 911.

What can you do about nighttime hypoglycemia?

The only sign that you have this problem may be elevated glucose levels in the morning or waking up drenched in sweat. You may also remember vivid dreams or nightmares and wake up with a headache in the morning. Checking your BG at 3:00 A.M. can detect middle-of-the-night lows. These may be eliminated by reducing your evening dose of NPH or lente or by changing the time you take it. If you take rapid-acting insulin at bedtime, reduce the dose. A snack at bedtime may help. Try one of the cornstarch-based bars made for this situation.

This chapter was written by Mark E. Molitch, MD.

3

Feet

Stop it at the start, it's late for medicine to be prepared
when disease has grown strong through long delays.
Ovid, 43 B.C.–17 A.D.
Remedia Amoris, 91

Case study

TJ is 62 years old and has had type 2 diabetes for 10 years. TJ
went walking on the beach with his grandchildren and cut his
foot on a seashell. He did not feel the cut, nor the sore that
developed. By the time he noticed redness and swelling, he
had walked on it for weeks, and it was infected. His doctor
has tried dressings and antibiotics, but the ulcer is not healing,
even though TJ still has good circulation in his feet. He is
afraid the front of his foot will have to be amputated.

Foot problems are one of the leading causes of hospitalization
for people with diabetes. The good news is that you can prevent most ulcers (and amputations) with daily foot inspections,
regular visits to your doctor and podiatrist, wearing proper
shoes, and finding problems early. The "stop it at the start"
philosophy is as practical today as it was in Ovid's time.

The foot is a marvelously intricate biomechanical structure
composed of 26 bones, 23 joints, and 42 muscles. When these

structures work together normally, your feet feel great. However, when they don't, serious problems can develop.

Is there one cause for the foot problems that lead to amputations?

Actually there are four: 1) nerve damage (loss of feeling), 2) poor circulation, 3) foot deformity, and 4) difficulty fighting infection. Add any injury to your "high risk foot" and you'll probably have an ulcer that is difficult to heal (Table 3-1).

Neuropathy

Nerve damage causes a loss of feeling in feet and legs. You may have numbness or tingling and not be able to feel where your feet are. We rely on pain to protect us from injury. If you buy a pair of new shoes and they rub a blister on your foot, you will stop wearing those shoes. If you can't feel the pain of

Table 3-1. Risk Factors for Diabetic Foot Ulcers

Within the Body Factors	Outside Factors
Neuropathy	Minor injury
Loss of feeling	High plantar pressures: callus build up
Muscle weakness	Shoe pressure: blisters
Vascular disease	Injury: cuts, lacerations, etc.
Poor circulation	Thermal injury
Difficulty healing	Burns from hot soaks, scalds, etc.
Poor response to infection	Frostbite
Foot deformity	Chemical burns: "corn cures"
Previous ulcer	Bathroom surgery on ingrown toenails, calluses, etc.
	Poor knowledge of diabetes
	Cigarette smoking

the blister, you keep on wearing them and do a lot of damage to your foot.

Neuropathy affects the nerves to the muscles in your feet and causes weakness and the development of hammertoes, bunions, or other deformities. When we walk, there is pressure on the bottom of our feet. With neuropathy, the bones on the bottom of the forefoot may shift position and increase the pressures on the skin beneath them, but you can't feel it. Continuing to walk on high pressure points breaks down the skin and causes ulcers.

Poor circulation

People with diabetes often have circulation problems in their feet due to atherosclerosis and blockage of arteries. Your feet may turn bright red when hanging down and constantly feel cold. Also, the skin may become shiny, thin, and easily damaged, and hair growth may be reduced. Reduced blood flow means your feet don't get enough oxygen or nutrients. When the foot is injured, infected, or ulcerated, healing will be slow or not happen at all.

Infection

People with diabetes are more likely to have infections, and their immune systems do not fight off infections well. Infections can rapidly worsen and go undetected, especially with nerve damage or poor circulation. The only sign of a developing infection may be unexplained high blood sugar levels.

If you have had a chronic foot ulcer for several months and suddenly develop a fever and flu-like symptoms, it may not be the flu; it may be spreading of the infection. Such infections must be treated with hospitalization and antibiotics to avoid gangrene. In fact, delaying treatment can make an amputation necessary.

Foot deformities

Foot deformities such as hammertoes and bunions are common but cause more problems for people with diabetes (Figure 3-1). These deformities can cause corns, calluses, blisters, and ulcers. A deformed foot requires a specially molded shoe. As Dr. Paul Brand said, "When a person with diabetes complains that his shoes are killing him, he may very well be correct."

How do foot deformities cause ulcers?

It isn't just that your shoes don't fit right. It's more a matter of your bones not being where they're supposed to be. Deformities of the foot and ankle cause increased pressure and irritation of the skin over the bumps and bony areas, causing damage leading to infection. Your earliest symptoms may be a slight reddening or thickening of the skin (corn or callus) beneath the ball of your foot or on your toes. You stress these areas every time you walk, and this may cause open sores and fractures.

What are some common foot deformities?

A hammertoe is a buckling of the toe, making it look like a swan's neck, that often occurs with a bunion. If you have diabetic neuropathy, hammertoes are often caused by weak muscles. The toe sits slightly back and up on the metatarsal head. This increases pressure on the ball of the foot, and shoes irritate the tip and top of the toe (Figure 3-1). Claw toes are similar to hammertoes but with more buckling (Figure 3-1). The toes sit on top of the metatarsal heads and push down on the ball of the foot, increasing pressure at that point. Claw toes usually are seen on feet with high arches, but not always.

The metatarsals are the five long bones in the middle of the foot just behind the toes. The metatarsal heads, which are similar to knuckles in the hand, are located in the ball of the foot

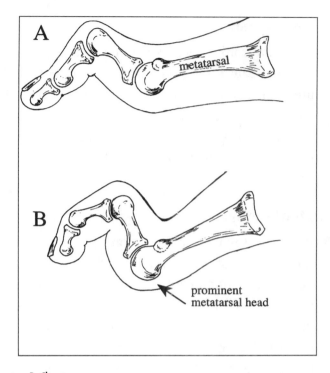

Figure 3-1. A. Hammertoe. B. Claw toe.
Reproduced with permission from Kelikian H: Deformities of the Lesser Toes, in Kelikian H, editor: *Hallux Valgus, Allied Deformities of the Forefoot and Metatarsalgia.* W. B. Saunders, 1965.

and support the body's weight. Normally, these bones share weight evenly. However, if one metatarsal bone is longer or lower than its neighbors, it carries too much weight. When you step on it, the high pressure on this point can cause pain, calluses, and ulcers.

A bunion is an enlarged bump at the big toe joint. Bunions are, most often, an inherited characteristic. The big toe angles toward the second toe and may underlap or override the second toe (Figure 3-2). When the foot is forced into a tight shoe, there is pressure over the bulge, which can result in an ulcer. Arthritis may be associated with bunions, with pain and stiffness of the joint. Restricted motion in the joint can cause a callus or ulcer beneath the big toe.

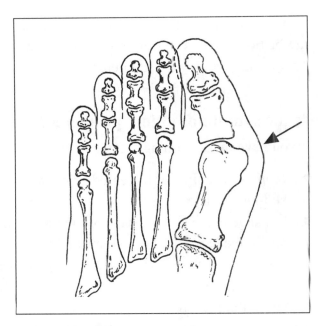

Figure 3-2. A bunion is a significant foot deformity.
Reproduced with permission from Kelikian H: Deformities of the Lesser Toes, in Kelikian H, editor: *Hallux Valgus, Allied Deformities of the Forefoot and Metatarsalgia.* W. B. Saunders, 1965.

What is Charcot's foot?

Charcot's (shar-kos) joints are not a common deformity, but they are serious. Most people go to their doctor because their foot is red and swollen, and their shoes don't fit. From this seemingly minor injury may come severe fractures and dislocations of joints in the foot and ankle. When the middle of the foot collapses, it causes a rocker-bottom shape to the foot and increased pressure on the bottom of the foot. This often results in ulcers. The foot can become so deformed that walking is difficult. Special footwear is very important for this condition.

People at high risk generally have had diabetes for more than 10 years, have loss of feeling in their feet, and are in their 50s or 60s. People who have complications affecting eyes, kidneys, and nerves appear to be at greatest risk. Injury to the foot can put you at risk, as does smoking, living alone, and not taking good care of your feet.

The treatment is to stop putting weight on the foot. This can be done by bed rest or with a special cast (p. 30). If you walk on it, you may cause fractures and more deformity.

What are the symptoms of foot problems?

If you have these warning signs, get prompt treatment:

- Redness, swelling, or increased skin temperature of the foot or ankle
- A change in the size or shape of the foot or ankle
- Pain in the legs at rest or while walking
- Open sores with or without drainage, no matter how small (ulcers)
- Nonhealing wounds
- Corns or calluses with skin discoloration

Are there treatments for foot deformities?

If you have foot deformities or a loss of feeling, you need therapeutic footwear (shoes, socks, and shoe inserts). All three work together to prevent ulcers. There are many types of shoes, socks, and inserts available. Your foot-care specialist can help you choose the ones that are correct for you. In some cases, especially when sores keep coming back, surgery might be an option.

What is an ulcer?

An ulcer is usually a painless open sore on the bottom of the foot or top of a toe. It results from pressure from your shoes, a corn or callus that has grown too thick, or an injury such as a splinter. Continued walking on the injury creates even further damage. The open sore frequently becomes infected and may even penetrate to the bone, even though you can only see a small sore on the surface of the skin.

How can ulcers be treated?

Find it early, see your doctor immediately, and don't walk on it. Your doctor will clean the wound, and apply dressings and give you antibiotics. All the dead tissue in an ulcer must be removed (debrided), so it will heal. The ulcer may need to be cultured for bacteria. X rays may help determine whether there is a foreign body in your foot, infection in the bone (osteomyelitis), or any gas or air deep in the tissues (which suggests infection). Sometimes, you need an examination using magnetic resonance imaging (MRI).

Proper wound care is important. There are many treatments for wounds, including saline, healing gels, ointments, and topical disinfectants or antibiotics. There are also many types of dressings to cover your wound, and different ones may be used at different points in the healing process. New products for wound healing include platelet-derived growth factors and tissue-engineered skin substitutes. They are not appropriate for all wounds, but they help heal better than standard saline dressings alone. Both deliver growth factors and live cells to your ulcer to speed up the healing.

Controlling your blood sugar is important because high blood sugar interferes with your white blood cells' ability to fight infection. Signs of the infection getting worse are increased redness around the ulcer or red streaks going up your leg. If you notice increased drainage and the foot has a bad odor, call your physician at once. If you develop pain or if the foot with an ulcer on the bottom gets red and puffy on the top, call your physician. These are signs of spreading infection. Do not soak your foot.

The most important thing you can do is to stay off the foot. Do not put weight on the ulcer. You may use crutches, a wheelchair, or bed rest. Special casts, braces, healing sandals, shoe inserts, or padding may also protect the foot while it heals.

How can you get around while the ulcer heals?

The best device for relieving pressure on an ulcer is a total contact cast or a non-weight-bearing removable cast. Many studies have shown that a total contact cast will heal 90–95% of wounds in an average of 6 weeks. A professional applies the cast, taking care to protect the skin from further injury. The cast protects the wound from the high pressures that caused it. It immobilizes the foot and helps control swelling, and it limits the amount of walking you can do. The cast is fairly heavy, may be hot, and cannot be removed for bathing. It is usually changed every 1–3 weeks. Your other option, a "clam shell" non-weight-bearing cast, can be removed at night and for bathing. But, it is expensive and cannot be adjusted to fit as the swelling goes down.

You might use a walker boot, which has a padded insert and padded uprights to protect the foot from high pressures. The soft insert spreads the pressures over a greater area of the foot. The walker boot can be removed to inspect the wound and for bathing. However, if you take the boot off and do any walking, even in the middle of the night to go to the bathroom, you can undo days of healing. It is not as heavy as a cast and is easier to put on and take off than a cast, but it may not be as effective in healing an ulcer.

Another choice is a half-shoe. It is lighter than a cast or boot, but it does relieve the pressure on the front part of the foot by forcing weight bearing onto the heel. The sole of the shoe ends before the forefoot, which can make walking difficult. You may need a cane or walker for balance. Healing time is not as fast as with a cast, but it's better than if you only wore therapeutic footwear.

Should you use a cane or walker with an ulcer?

A cane, crutches, or a walker can help unload pressure from the foot even further when you use them with casts, boots, or shoes. Any pressure taken by the arms is weight that doesn't have to go through the feet. Use them if you feel more stable; don't if you don't. It's up to you and your doctor.

What shoes should you wear after the ulcer is healed?

After your wound is healed, your foot is even more likely to develop an ulcer than before. You need to check your feet very carefully every day. Even though the ulcer has healed on the surface, you will wear a walker boot for several weeks or months as the skin gets stronger. Your doctor will refer you to a pedorthist for special shoes to protect your feet (p. 41).

Why don't some ulcers heal?

Ulcers can take months to heal. During this time, try to keep your diabetes in good control to encourage healing. When ulcers are slow to heal or get worse, you have to consider the possible causes. First, some people don't stay off the foot. If walking or weight bearing is the cause of the ulcer, it makes sense that continued walking will prevent it from healing. (You do not cure tennis elbow by continuing to play tennis!) Denial is common, because people with neuropathy can't feel pain. If it doesn't hurt, it is easy to ignore. Walking continues (without a limp), the pressure continues, and the ulcer cannot heal. Also, many people can't take time off from their jobs to heal. Wheelchairs, crutches, or casts can help.

A second reason the ulcer won't heal can be poor circulation, which prevents the blood from delivering nutrients, oxygen, and antibiotics to the ulcer. Without adequate blood flow to the foot, the ulcer will not heal. Your physician can check blood pressure at your ankles and arms. It should be the same, and if it is not, you may have blocked arteries. When significant blockages exist, you may be referred to a vascular surgeon. Bypass operations in the legs and feet can restore circulation and promote healing of ulcers (chapter 10).

Deep-seated infection is the third major reason many foot ulcers do not heal. Chronic infections often have no symptoms. Constant draining or a discharge from the ulcer may be a sign of an underlying infection. Wound cultures are taken periodically to check the bacterial growth in the ulcer and to determine which, if any, of the bacteria need to be treated with antibiotics. Keep in mind, however, that cultures taken by swabbing may not yield the bacteria that is actually causing the infection. Antibiotic treatment based on the false culture results may not help. Tissue obtained from debridement or a punch biopsy may be sent for analysis. If a probe can actually touch bone at the base of the ulcer, it strongly suggests bone infection (osteomyelitis) that will require more aggressive treatment. Periodic X rays will show any underlying bone changes. If you have a long-standing ulcer that suddenly gets worse, with fever and elevated blood sugar levels, you need immediate hospitalization.

How can you prevent an ulcer from developing?

Prevention is the key. Develop good habits and continue them for your lifetime. Use the "5 Ps" of prevention: professional care, protective footwear, pressure reduction, preventive surgery, and preventive education (Table 3-2).

Professional care

You need regular examinations by a health care professional familiar with diabetic foot care. For example, your diabetes doctor can examine your feet and check for neuropathy, circulation problems, and potential trouble spots. A podiatrist can also check your feet and trim toenails and calluses before they become problems. Studies have shown that such regular care—at least several times each year—is important in preventing foot problems, especially if you have neuropathy.

Table 3-2. The 5 Ps of Prevention

1. Professional care

>Regular visits, examinations, and foot care

>Early detection and aggressive treatment of new ulcers

2. Protective shoes

>Well cushioned walking shoes

>Extra-depth or custom-molded shoes

3. Pressure reduction

>Cushioned insoles, custom orthotics, padded socks

>Pressure measurements, computerized or mat

4. Preventive surgery

>Correct hammertoes, bunions, Charcot's joint, etc.

>Prevent ulcers over or under deformities from reappearing

5. Preventive education

>Patient education: need for daily inspection and early treatment

>Physician education: significance of foot ulcers, importance of regular foot examinations, and current diabetic foot management

Protective footwear

Many of the minor injuries leading to foot ulcers are caused by poorly fitting shoes. A professional should assist you in selecting and fitting shoes for the shape of your foot and any deformity you have. Walking or athletic shoes are good for most everyone; but studies have shown that people with a healed ulcer who wore specially designed shoes (with extra depth for the toes and cushioned soles) were much less likely to get another ulcer than were people who continued to wear their regular shoes.

Pressure reduction

You can relieve pressure on the soles of your feet by wearing cushioned shoes, padded socks, and insoles. The most com-

mon sign of higher-than-normal pressures on the foot is a callus, which is the skin's normal response to excessive pressure.
If you reduce the pressure on this part of the foot, you can
reduce the size of the callus and possibly prevent an ulcer
from developing under it. Most ulcers occur where there is a
callus. If the callus comes back after the ulcer heals, there is a
strong likelihood the ulcer will come back, too.

High pressures can be measured by footprint analysis using
pressure-sensitive mats or by computerized gait analysis systems. Potential problem areas or "hot spots" can be detected
and treated with inserts for your shoes. In-shoe pressure measurements are useful for seeing how well the insoles work.

Preventive surgery

Occasionally, foot surgery stops ulcers by repairing a deformity in the foot that would eventually cause an ulcer. Recon-
structive surgery is often necessary to heal chronic ulcers that
don't respond to other treatments. This does not mean that you
need a routine correction of any hammertoe or foot deformity.
Most are best managed by special shoes and pressure-
reduction therapies. The decision to have surgery must be a
joint one made by you, your family, your primary physician,
and the surgeon. Avoid unnecessary surgery at all costs. This
surgery is done only in people with healthy arteries, and
requires good post-operative care to be successful.

Preventive education

Many foot ulcers are caused by poor self-care or neglect. You
need to know what to do. That is why foot-care education from
your diabetes educator, nurse specialist, physician, or podiatrist
is so valuable. Foot care is seldom accomplished by one health
care provider. You usually will have a team, depending on the
condition of your feet. Nothing is more important than keeping
your feet clean and dry and inspecting them every day.

Remove both shoes and socks at every doctor's appointment. Take part in diabetic foot-care courses, and learn to recognize warning signs. That's how you reduce your risk for foot ulcers.

Who should see your feet?

Foot problems may require care from your primary care physician, an endocrinologist or diabetologist, a podiatrist, an orthopedic surgeon, a plastic surgeon, a vascular surgeon, a diabetes educator, a wound-care specialist, or a rehabilitation specialist experienced in the management of people with diabetes. These team members should communicate with each other about your condition and treatment.

What type of shoes should you wear?

You can buy shoes off the shelf or have them custom made, but in any case, the shoes are meant to protect your feet, not to hurt them. Shoes made of leather easily adapt to the shape of your feet and allow your feet to breathe. Athletic shoes, jogging shoes, and sneakers are excellent choices as long as they fit well and provide adequate cushioning.

If you can, change your shoes several times a day so that one pair is not worn for more than 4–6 hours. Only wear new shoes a few hours at a time, and then inspect your feet for redness or irritation.

Above all, do not walk barefooted. Discuss wearing open-toed shoes or sandals with your podiatrist or physician. At the beach or pool, wear water shoes, especially if you have lost feeling in your feet.

What features should you look for in a shoe?

Make sure the shoes are the kind called in-depth or extra-depth shoes. In-depth shoes have 1/4–1/2 inch more room from top to bottom in the toe box than a regular shoe (Figure 3-3). They usually also have a removable insole that

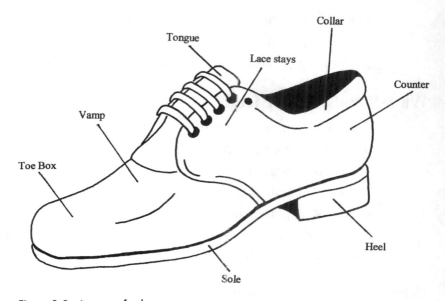

Figure 3-3. Anatomy of a shoe.

can be taken out for more room, or to make room for a special shoe insert. These shoes are great for accommodating foot deformities or shoe inserts. They can also help prevent deformities, such as hammertoes and bunions.

Steer clear of slip-on shoes, which are generally too tight and often too short. They are designed this way because if they truly fit the shape of your foot, they'd keep falling off. Shoes that tie or have velcro are best. You can loosen them as the day goes on, especially if your feet and ankles swell. Shoes that tie put less pressure on your forefoot and can prevent the development of blisters or calluses.

Look for shoes that come in a variety of widths—narrow, medium, wide, and extra wide. Some shoe manufacturers use letters: A means narrow and E means wide.

All feet are shaped differently, as are all shoes. The important thing is getting a good match. It's best to find a shoe that resembles the shape of your foot. Try to avoid shoes that have pointed toes, which cramp your toes and bend them into

unnatural positions. A shoe with a broad, rounded toe is best
(Figure 3-4).

High heels are another thing to avoid. The higher the heel,
the more pressure there is on the ball of the foot and toes.
High heels are especially bad when they are combined with a
pointed toe box, as in cowboy boots and women's shoes.

The soles of your shoes are important to consider. Thick,
cushioned wedge soles are appropriate for most people. A
wedge sole is flat along the entire bottom of the shoe, with no
separate heel. Dense foam rubber soles offer more cushioning
than leather soles. Shoes with built in rocker soles decrease
the pressures under the ball of the foot, helping to prevent
ulcers. You can have rocker soles put on most any shoe if you
need them (Figure 3-5).

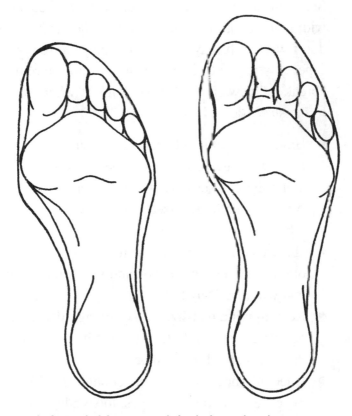

Figure 3-4. The foot on the left is not properly fit. The foot on the right is.

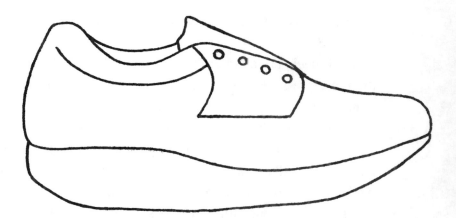

Figure 3-5. Rocker sole shoe.

How do you know if your shoes fit?

Shoes must always fit comfortably, with adequate length, width, and depth for your toes. If a shoe is hard to put on, don't wear it. It may be too small and cause serious damage, especially if you have neuropathy or poor circulation. Don't "break in" new shoes: If they don't fit when you try them on in the store, don't buy them.

- Have your feet sized every time you buy shoes. Your feet tend to get longer and wider as you grow older. You might be surprised to find what your size is now. And have both feet sized—one may be longer than the other.
- Have your feet measured at the end of the day. Feet often swell during the day, and you want to buy shoes that will fit *all* day long.
- Keep in mind that sizes vary among different shoe brands and styles. Judge the shoe by how it fits, not by the size marked in the shoe.
- Once the shoes are on, there should be 3/8 to 1/2 inch of space beyond your longest toe while you're

standing; at the same time, the ball of your foot should fit well into the widest part of the shoe. Always try on shoes with the socks on that you will wear with them.

● Walk in the shoes to make sure they fit well. The heels should not slip very much.

A qualified shoe fitter measures your feet with a Bannock device, to get the length from heel to toe, from heel to ball, and width, to be sure that your shoes are not too tight, causing pressure, nor too loose, causing shear.

You should be able to pinch some leather between your fingers across the top of the shoe, or vamp. Properly fitting shoes will tend to slip a little in the heel. No slippage indicates that the shoe is too short. If you have shoe inserts, try them on with your new shoes. They will change the fit.

Will the shoes be ugly?

Most therapeutic shoes nowadays don't look like the orthopedic shoes of the past. They can be walking or running shoes, work boots, or hiking boots. You can even get dress shoes (the policy for wearing dress shoes, however, is like the one for dessert—not very much and not very often). The shoes can be very attractive. In fact, unless your feet have severe deformities requiring custom shoes, no one will even know that you are wearing special shoes.

What kind of socks should you wear?

White socks are preferred so you can see blood, for example from a blister. Look for socks made of materials that wick moisture away from the skin, such as CoolMAX or Duraspun. These socks, made of acrylic fibers, are bulkier and provide more cushioning and less friction. There are socks for people with diabetes that don't have seams, wick moisture away, and have special cushioning under the ball of the foot and the heel.

What will shoe inserts do for your feet?

Shoe inserts (also called orthotics or arch supports) cushion and protect your feet. They off-load high pressure in specific areas on the bottoms of your feet by distributing your weight equally over the entire soles of your feet. They are also used to correct the position of your feet or to provide pain relief.

How do you obtain shoe inserts?

Your physician refers you to a specialist to make molds of your feet to make the inserts. A certified pedorthist is the most qualified person, in this situation, to make foot orthotics. Your doctor may refer you to a certified orthotist, who has had special training in providing braces and supports for the entire body, including the feet. In any case, you will need a prescription. If you have lost feeling in your feet, have diabetes, and have a foot deformity or have had a foot ulcer, Medicare and many health insurance companies will pay for up to 80% of custom footwear.

What are the types of shoe inserts?

Some inserts are made of soft, lightweight foam. They don't last long, but they offer the best cushioning. They are often bulky and some people need a larger shoe to use them. Weight-distributing inserts commonly have a soft foam layer on top (next to your foot) and a firmer material, such as cork, underneath. This type of insert offers you cushioning and protection while equalizing pressures on the bottoms of your feet. Sometimes a shock-absorbing material is included. These are full-length inserts. This type of insert routinely wears out after a year or two, but it should be checked by your pedorthist every six months or so.

A functional shoe insert is made of a thin, rigid plastic that runs from the heel to the ball of your foot. If your health care team asks for it, a soft topcover can be applied. The plastic base of this insert lasts for years, but the topcover will need to be replaced periodically.

It's rare, but sometimes, an over-the-counter shoe insert works. Custom-made devices can be costly, and some insurance plans do not pay for them, so an over-the-counter device can be a lower-cost alternative. However, you must have no deformities or nerve damage. And you may need them to be customized for you.

Where can you buy therapeutic shoes?

Specialty shoe stores or comfort shoe stores are better equipped to help you than a large discount shoe store or a department store. Some stores specialize in walking shoes and therapeutic shoes and may have a certified pedorthist on staff. Certified pedorthists are trained in foot anatomy and the construction of shoes, shoe modifications, and foot orthotics (inserts). Like a pharmacist, a pedorthist fills the prescription for therapeutic shoes that was written for you. Check out the store thoroughly, because this is likely to be a long-term relationship. There may also be pedorthic facilities near you. They have pedorthists on staff and stock a more specialized inventory of shoes.

About 85% of people can be fitted with off-the-shelf shoes. Off-the-shelf shoes may need some adjustment to fit your needs. The uppers may need to be stretched for prominent toes, wedges and flares can be added to the soles for better stability, and rocker soles or metatarsal bars can be added to reduce pressure on certain areas of the foot. Shoes with laces can be converted to Velcro closure if needed. Lifts are added to the inside or outside of the shoes if your legs are different lengths. If your feet can't fit into standard footwear, the pedorthist can fit you for custom-made shoes. These take 3–6 weeks to make.

What sort of follow-up do you have with special shoes?

Your shoes and shoe inserts should be checked by your pedorthist or orthotist every six months. When you get shoes and inserts, your practitioner will tell you how long it will take to break them in. There will be a few scheduled follow-up appointments during the first month or two, but then you are on your own. Most facilities send you a reminder about setting up a visit every six months, but it is your responsibility to make sure your shoes and inserts are working properly. If you develop any red spots, blisters, calluses or other pain, make an appointment to see your health care team, pedorthist, or orthotist immediately.

Will your insurance pay for therapeutic shoes?

In 1995, legislation was passed called the Therapeutic Shoe Bill (TSB). The TSB provides a special exception for people with diabetes to get coverage for their shoes and inserts, because Medicare does not normally pay for shoes and/or inserts. There are several points that you will need to know regarding the TSB.

Only people with diabetes are eligible for the benefits under the TSB. You also need to have another qualifying complication, such as an ulcer or a thick callus, a history of ulcers, deformity in your feet, loss of feeling, or poor circulation. The physician managing your diabetes must certify that you have diabetes and have foot complications. There is a standard form for your physician to fill out before you can get your shoes and inserts, and a prescription is required as well.

A facility that is either a registered Medicare provider or a registered Medicare supplier must be used. A Medicare provider performs the service and then bills Medicare directly. A Medicare supplier has you pay up front, and then submits a claim to Medicare, so you are reimbursed for the amount that Medicare allows for the services provided.

The TSB covers in-depth shoes and shoe inserts. The shoes can be either off-the-shelf or custom made, but the inserts must be specifically designed for your feet, not just ones purchased over-the-counter.

One pair of shoes per calendar year and up to three pairs of inserts are covered. Modifications to shoes, such as rocker soles, can be substituted for inserts. Medicare covers 80% of the allowable costs for these goods. If you have supplemental insurance, it will often cover the other 20%.

Call your insurance plan's customer service center and verify whether they cover therapeutic footwear. Unfortunately, many health insurance carriers do not recognize how important therapeutic footwear is and will not pay for these services.

How should I care for my foot after an amputation?

Amputation can "create" a foot deformity, and put unusual pressure on the bones in the foot. Although the surgery may be necessary to save the foot, it increases the risk for future ulcers and amputation. You will need padding in your shoe and well-fitting therapeutic shoes.

If you ever have an amputation, give yourself time to adjust. Physical therapy can help with strength and mobility. You may be surprised, however, by the emotions you feel. Talking with a counselor or a support group can help you regain your emotional balance, too.

What are the guidelines for good foot care?

- At each doctor's visit, remove your shoes and stockings, and have your feet examined.
- Don't walk barefoot.
- Look inside your shoes for sharp tacks, rough linings, or foreign objects before you put them on.
- Wear sensible shoes that are properly fitted.
- Inspect your feet daily for blisters, bleeding, and sores between toes. Make this part of your ritual.

- Use a long-handled mirror to see the bottom of your foot and heel. Ask a family member for help if you can't see well.
- Do not soak your feet.
- Don't use hot water bottles, heating pads, or electric blankets on your feet. Test bath water with your elbow.
- Wash feet daily with warm, soapy water and dry them well, especially between the toes. Put on clean socks.
- Use moisturizing lotion (whose first ingredient is not alcohol) daily but not between the toes.
- Do not use acids or chemical corn removers.
- Do not perform "bathroom surgery" on corns, calluses, or ingrown toenails.
- Trim your nails long and following the curve of the toe. If necessary, file them gently. Have a podiatrist do this if you have difficulty doing it, and especially if you have neuropathy.
- Call your doctor immediately if your foot becomes swollen, red, or painful. Stay off the foot.
- Don't smoke.
- Learn all you can about diabetes and foot care.
- Have regular foot examinations by your physician or podiatrist.

Robert G. Frykberg, DPM, MPH; Lee J. Sanders, DPM; Erick Janisse, CPed, BOCO; Michael J. Mueller, PT, PhD; and David R. Sinacore, PT, PhD, contributed to this chapter.

4

Eye Disease

Case study

A 36-year-old man who has had type 1 diabetes for 18 years awakened with blurred vision. Six months ago, he noted a web in front of one eye, but it cleared in a few days. It happened again, 6 weeks ago, and lasted 1 week. When questioned, he realizes he now has difficulty with depth perception such as when attempting to add cream to his coffee.

The ophthalmologist explains the sudden onset of floating specks may be a harmless change in the vitreous gel, the material that fills the globe of the eye. However, in a diabetic patient, there is a possibility the floating specks may be caused by a hemorrhage. The doctor will do a dilated-eye exam to evaluate the retina and vitreous gel.

Case study

A 60-year-old woman with a 12-year history of type 2 diabetes reports the gradual onset of blurred vision. She has difficulty completing tasks at work, and her employer has complained that she makes too many mistakes. Stronger reading glasses no longer help. A dilated-eye exam will show any signs of retinopathy and whether a cataract is present. Examination of her macula with a special lens determines that she has macular swelling.

Introduction

Diabetes can affect your eyes and vision. Some of these effects are mild or short term, such as the blurred vision that comes with poor blood glucose control. Certain complications, however, can be sight threatening, even when your vision is normal. Diabetes is the leading cause of new-onset legal blindness in the U.S. Most of this blindness can be prevented if you keep your blood sugar levels close to normal and if you receive regular examinations and prompt treatment by a physician with experience in diabetic eye care. Because there is usually no pain associated with diabetic eye disease, most people do not have their eyes examined as often as they should.

Regular, life-long eye care is one of the most important elements of managing your diabetes. **Visit an eye-care specialist at least once a year even if your vision hasn't changed**. When diabetic eye disease is caught early, treatment can be very successful. Current treatments such as laser surgery can prevent more than 95% of severe vision loss from proliferative diabetic retinopathy (disease of the retina) and more than 50% of moderate vision loss from diabetic macular edema (swelling of the macula, a part of the retina).

How do you see?

Your vision is a highly developed and complex process. For you to be able to see, light must be focused by the cornea and lens of the eye through the vitreous gel that fills the eye and onto the retina in the back of the eye, where it is changed into signals that are carried along nerve fibers within the eye (Figure 4-1). These signals are transmitted through the optic nerve to a rear portion of the brain called the visual cortex. Here, visual signals are processed by the brain as sight. Nerves also control the movement of your eyes, adjust the focus, or alter pupil size.

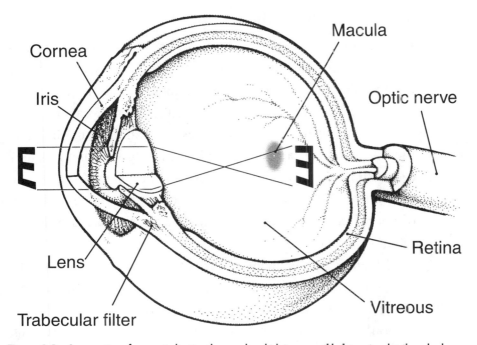

Cornea

Iris

Macula

Optic nerve

Lens

Trabecular filter

Retina

Vitreous

Figure 4-1. Cross-section of an eye indicating the macula, which is responsible for seeing details and color vision.

Any abnormality in the visual system can interfere with your ability to see. For clear vision, there must be no obstruction along the light path within the eye. Scars on the cornea, imperfections in the lens of the eye (such as cataracts), or cloudiness in the vitreous gel of the eye can interfere with light focusing on the retina. The retina is very important to vision. It must be healthy and have a good blood supply, and the nerve transmissions to the brain must go smoothly. The retina can be divided into two zones. The *macula*, or center of the retina, is responsible for detailed central vision that allows you to read, recognize faces, drive, and distinguish colors. The remaining areas of the retina provide peripheral (side) vision, motion detection, and night vision. Obviously, any disease that affects your retina affects your vision.

How does diabetes affect the retina?

Damage to the retina from diabetes is called *diabetic retinopathy*. The retina consists of many small blood vessels—and uncontrolled blood glucose levels damage small blood vessels. In the eye, this damage changes blood flow and weakens blood vessel walls. The vessel walls can balloon out, allowing fluid or blood to leak into the retina, causing swelling (edema) or bleeding (hemorrhages). This is called *nonproliferative* retinopathy. The retina gets less blood and oxygen. This loss of nourishment is called *ischemia*. The affected areas of the retina stop working.

If there is no treatment at this point, the eye will attempt to compensate. The retina will release growth factors that cause new blood vessels to grow on the retina or on the optic nerve. Although this may seem logical, it often results in devastating complications. The growth of new blood vessels is called *proliferative retinopathy*. The abnormal new vessels are fragile and will bleed and leak. They do not nourish the areas of the eye that have lost circulation and serve no useful purpose.

New blood vessels growing between the retina and the vitreous gel get pulled and tend to hemorrhage or leak into the gel. The vitreous gel naturally contracts with aging, but this happens earlier in people with diabetes. If the vitreous detaches before retinopathy develops, you may see a floating line or web, particularly when looking at a bright background, and flashes of light often seen at night. If proliferative retinopathy has begun, the separation of the vitreous gel breaks the blood vessels. Blood flowing into the vitreous gel blocks the path of light, causing you to see floaters, which may vary from a few specks to a dark spot that blocks most of your vision. (Not all floaters indicate proliferative retinopathy.)

Without treatment at this point, scar tissue can develop along with these vessels and, as they contract, can pull on the retina and cause it to detach. The visual receptors (rods and cones) in the retina stop working when they are separated from the cells beneath them. Zones that have been detached show up as blanks in your field of vision.

What is macular edema?

Fluid leaking into the tissues of the retina causes swelling (edema). Leakage that settles in the macula area of the retina is called *diabetic macular edema* (DME). Edema that involves or threatens the center of the macula is called *clinically significant macular edema* (CSME). The macula is responsible for detailed vision, so you may experience visual blur for both near and distant objects. Diabetic macular edema can sometimes cause you to be less sensitive to blue and yellow colors.

A person with uncontrolled type 2 diabetes is especially likely to develop macular edema. Because many people have type 2 diabetes, macular edema accounts for most of the cases of vision loss from diabetes.

What puts you at risk for developing retinopathy?

How long you have had diabetes, your level of blood glucose control, and other medical conditions—such as hypertension, kidney disease, high cholesterol and other blood fat levels, and pregnancy—put you at risk for diabetic retinopathy. People with high blood glucose levels are more likely to develop retinopathy.

If you have type 2 diabetes, you might have had some level of retinopathy when you were diagnosed, because most people with type 2 diabetes have had it for awhile before they are diagnosed. You should have yearly eye examinations, because retinopathy can occur any time after diagnosis.

What are the symptoms of retinopathy?

You may have serious, sight-threatening retinopathy even though you have no symptoms, and vision can measure even better than 20/20 (normal vision). For this reason, annual eye examinations are so important. An exam for glasses or a change in your old prescription is not enough. You need a detailed examination of both the retina and the lens. Ophthalmologists and some optometrists are skilled in this exam. However, some optometrists do not do this dilated-eye examination, so make sure that you ask.

Symptoms of changes in your retinas may include blurred or fluctuating vision, floating spots, warping of straight lines, or loss of vision. Distortion of straight lines can be a serious symptom. Many patients first notice it while observing tiles or floor patterns with one eye closed. This distortion is often a sign of macular edema. Floating spots may be the result of age-related changes, but they may also indicate vitreous hemorrhage. A blockage of vision that is like a window shade being drawn across your field of view may indicate retinal detachment. With any symptom, play it safe, and have your eyes examined.

What happens at your eye examination?

You need to see an eye-care specialist experienced in managing diabetic eye disease, an ophthalmologist or specially trained optometrist. This examination should include measurement of your level of vision, evaluation of the movement of your eyes, refraction to determine your need for glasses, glaucoma screening, cataract evaluation, evaluation of changes in color perception or night vision, and dilation of your pupils to examine your retinas. Examination of the retina to detect retinopathy may require different techniques from those used in a routine eye examination. The eye-care specialist needs to be able to see your entire retina and vitreous gel.

The eye-care specialist may use a handheld ophthalmoscope, an indirect ophthalmoscope worn on his or her head, and/or the slit-lamp biomicroscope. The handheld ophthalmoscope gives a magnified view of the optic nerve head, macula, and blood vessels of the retina.

You rest your chin on the slit-lamp biomicroscope while the eye-care specialist uses different lenses to examine the vitreous gel and retina. Occasionally, during this part of the examination, your eye may be anesthetized with drops, and a contact lens may be used.

Your pupil dilation and eye examination cause no harm to the retina. After the examination, you may have temporary dim vision or see various colors. Because of the pupil dilation, your vision may seem blurry for several hours, particularly for close-up work, and you are likely to be sensitive to light.

Are there other tests for diagnosing retinopathy?

Other diagnostic techniques that may be useful include fluorescein dye angiography and ultrasonography.

Fluorescein angiography

Fluorescein angiography is a technique in which pictures are taken of the retina while a fluorescent dye is flowing through its blood vessels. It requires an intravenous injection of the dye (usually in your arm) and a complex camera and lighting system. Details of the retinal circulation, including the smallest blood vessels, known as capillaries, can be evaluated by this technique. A series of up to 36 slides are taken to record the dye flow. Vessels that are healthy prevent the dye from leaking through the blood vessel walls. Vessels that are diseased allow the dye to leak. An accumulation of dye in the retina is a sign of edema. Areas of reduced blood flow can also be seen.

This is a diagnostic test only; it is not a treatment. Following the test, you may notice your vision is temporarily blurred or dimmed, or you may see peculiar colors for a few moments. Vision rapidly returns to its pretest condition. You may notice a slight yellow or tan appearance to your skin and to the whites of your eyes lasting approximately 24 hours. The injected dye is cleared rapidly by way of the urinary system, giving a peculiar color to your urine. However, this dye can be safely used even in patients who have diabetic kidney disease, including patients who require dialysis.

You should be aware that the injection of any medicine or dye can be associated with complications, including allergic reactions. Fortunately, however, these are uncommon with fluorescein angiography. When the dye is first injected, you might feel a sensation of nausea that typically lasts only a few seconds. This is not an allergic reaction and should not prevent you from having future testing. The few patients who do suffer an allergic reaction to the fluorescein dye usually experience itching of their skin due to hives and rarely suffer a severe shocklike reaction. Patients who are allergic to the dye may, in fact, be able to undergo a future dye test with appropriate preoperative medications and careful medical supervision.

Angiography is used to determine the extent of background retinopathy and the points of leakage. These changes in the retina cannot be measured as well just by looking, and the angiogram helps to locate precise areas that require treatment. The physician can also see whether there is impairment of the circulation of the macula, which is so vital to your sight. Angiography is not routinely used to detect proliferative retinopathy, except when hidden zones of blood vessel growth are suspected.

Ultrasonography

Using sound waves, ultrasound builds a picture of an area of the body that cannot be observed directly. It is a method for evaluating the back portion of the eye in people who have obstructions in the eye, such as advanced cataracts or hemorrhage in the vitreous gel. It may allow the physician to discover a retinal detachment or scar tissue on the surface of the retina. It does not provide a view of the retina itself. Again, the ultrasound study is a method to diagnose and understand retinal anatomy and disease. Ultrasonography is particularly helpful in patients who have chronic vitreous hemorrhage and is often used before vitrectomy surgery.

There are other tests, including optical coherence tomography, which uses ultrasound to measure the thickness of the retina and can give an indication of the degree of edema in a patient with nonproliferative (background) retinopathy. Such techniques have only recently been developed, and although promising, their use is not yet widespread.

What is the treatment for nonproliferative retinopathy?

Controlling blood glucose and blood pressure are the keys to treating diabetic eye disease. Treatment of nonproliferative retinopathy may involve the use of lasers to seal the places that are leaking or to make it easier for the retina to absorb the leakage. A fluorescein angiogram can be used to map areas that require treatment. New zones of leakage may develop. That is why you may require a series of treatments.

Nonproliferative retinopathy is classified as mild, moderate, severe, or very severe. The level of retinopathy indicates the risk of your eye progressing to sight-threatening proliferative retinopathy and determines how often you need to have eye examinations. Ask your eye doctor what level of retinopathy you have and to send a letter to your diabetes care provider. It is not enough to be told, "You have some eye changes, come back in a few months."

What is the treatment for proliferative retinopathy?

Proliferative retinopathy is treated with lasers, cryotherapy (freezing), and vitrectomy (removal of vitreous gel). The choice of which to use depends on several factors. Some people have proliferative retinopathy only. Others have a combination of macular swelling and proliferation. Some patients may have hemorrhage, and others may have scar tissue pulling on the retina. Some patients may have cataracts obscuring the view of the retina. Occasionally, patients have new vessel growth on the iris as well, threatening to cause neovascular glaucoma. Each factor must be weighed by the ophthalmologist to determine the best course of management.

Laser treatment

The treatment for proliferative retinopathy is designed to stop the abnormal blood vessels from growing, bleeding, and contracting. Laser is used to destroy the ischemic areas of the retina that cause new blood vessels to grow. Destruction of these tissues causes the existing abnormal blood vessels to atrophy and prevents the growth of new blood vessels.

Laser also can be used to destroy abnormal blood vessels depending on their location. If the blood vessels are on the surface of the retina away from the macula and limited in size, they can be directly treated with the laser. This is called *a local laser treatment*. Local laser surgery is rarely performed alone, but usually along with scatter laser surgery.

If the blood vessels are on the optic nerve surface, direct laser surgery could damage the optic nerve. For vessels on the nerve or elsewhere, the method is to scatter treatment throughout the retina to destroy the unhealthy zones. Treatment not only stops production of growth factors but also may increase the amount of oxygen getting to the remaining retina. The end result is to cut back the new blood vessels without using laser directly on the optic nerve head or the abnormal blood vessels themselves. The scatter treatment involves approximately 1,200 to 1,800 laser applications in the midperipheral and peripheral (side) retina. The treatment is usually applied over two or three sessions. If all scatter laser surgery is applied in one session, it might cause excessive swelling in the retina and lead to macular edema, changes in vision, and, in rare cases, angle-closure glaucoma.

Laser surgery is generally performed in the ophthalmologist's office as an outpatient procedure. The eye is anesthetized with an eyedrop. A contact lens is placed on the eye, similar to the lens used for retinal examination. This lens holds your eyelid open and focuses the laser light. The laser applications are usually placed in rapid sequence, since less precise location is necessary. The ophthalmologist avoids large blood vessels, areas of hemorrhage, and the macula. Possible side effects of scatter laser treatment include decreased night vision and some loss of peripheral vision. Sometimes laser treatments can alter color vision. Local laser surgery involves fewer laser applications (usually fewer than 100), but the applications are placed much more precisely. Consequently, it will take more time between applications as the ophthalmologist focuses the laser in precise position.

The physician usually treats the lower portion of the retina first, so that any bleeding would settle in the region of the retina that has already been treated. This would allow the physician to see clearly to complete the treatment to the top portion of the retina. Depending on the degree of treatment required, one or more sessions may be necessary.

For patients who also have macular edema, it is desirable to treat the swelling first and then do the scatter treatment for the proliferative retinopathy. The goal is to reduce the swelling because scatter treatment may also cause swelling. In this instance, points of leakage surrounding the macula get local treatment. Then, in multiple sessions, scatter treatment can be done to the overgrowth of blood vessels.

In patients who have scar tissue on the retina, the ophthalmologist may need multiple sessions to avoid the areas of scar tissue and prevent contracting them further.

Patients with a cataract may present a challenge because the cataract may prevent examination of the retina and block the laser from reaching the retina. Occasionally, it is necessary to do cataract surgery first to be able to see and treat the retina. However, physicians generally prefer to treat the retina before doing cataract surgery and then evaluate the eye once again after the cataract has been removed.

For patients who also have a vitreous hemorrhage, laser treatment may be difficult to do. Patients with such hemorrhages are advised to sleep with the head of the bed elevated and to avoid bending with their head below the heart so that gravity will help the hemorrhage to settle in the lower portion of the eye. Not exercising may also help the hemorrhage to settle and allow the ophthalmologist to examine and treat the upper portions of the retina. As the hemorrhage settles, more of the retina becomes visible, and the scatter treatment can be completed. The image you see is reversed by the eye, so if you have a hemorrhage that settles in the bottom of your eye, you will see the floating debris at the top of your field of vision.

Cryotherapy

Cryotherapy (freezing) is sometimes used for the management of proliferative retinopathy. It allows treatment of the far edges of the retina that are hard to reach by laser. Cryotherapy has been used in patients who previously have had complete laser treatment but still have new blood vessel growth and bleeding. Vitrectomy is more common today. Cryotherapy may be useful in individuals who have hemorrhage that prevents the laser treatment and are not candidates for vitrectomy.

Vitrectomy

For the few patients who have chronic vitreous hemorrhage that does not go away or for patients with hemorrhages in both eyes who cannot carry out their normal daily functions such as eating, dressing, or taking medications, vitrectomy surgery may be indicated. A hemorrhage on the surface of the retina that blocks the macula is often a reason for vitrectomy surgery because such hemorrhages tend to go away slowly and may result in the formation of scar tissue that covers the macula and pulls on the retina. Scar tissue pulling on the retina can be another reason for vitrectomy.

What happens in laser surgery?

Lasers create thin beams of light of differing wavelengths or colors. Ophthalmic lasers creating green, red, yellow, or infrared wavelengths can be used to clot leaking blood vessels, destroy zones of overgrown blood vessels, or destroy zones of ischemic retina. The laser light penetrates the eye; travels through the aqueous, lens, and vitreous; and is absorbed in the deepest layers of the retina, where the light energy is converted to heat. The heat burns and seals the surrounding area, which heals as a laser scar.

Different wavelengths of light may serve useful purposes. For instance, red wavelengths penetrate blood in the vitreous or a cataract better than green wavelengths. The photoreceptors (rods and cones) in the areas that are treated are destroyed by the treatment, and thus laser scars are typically blank spots in the field of vision. These blank spots generally don't bother you because they are tiny and located away from the central area responsible for detail vision.

Anesthesia

The need for anesthesia varies. It is important for you to remain still during treatment. Most patients do this by staring at a target with the eye that is not being treated while the other eye is being treated. If you cannot remain still or if anesthetic drops in your eyes are not enough, then a local anesthesia by injection into the tissues surrounding the eye is used. Some cases require treatment extraordinarily close to the center of the macula, the most visually sensitive zone of the retina. In these cases, the physician may choose to immobilize your eye by injecting a local anesthetic into the tissues around the eye. As a rule, laser treatment causes very little discomfort. However, depending on the amount of treatment required or depending on specific regions of the retina that need treatment, some patients may experience localized discomfort during treatment or a posttreatment headache.

Laser surgery procedure

You are seated and rest your chin and forehead in a stabilizing device. You get an anesthetic eyedrop and then a contact lens is put in position on the surface of your cornea. The physician may project photographic images of the retina or of the fluorescein angiogram to use as a map to locate the points that require treatment. The physician will choose the appropriate wavelength of light for your retina. The laser typically emits a very-low-power aiming beam that the physician can direct to the point needing treatment. When the laser is fired, that aiming beam becomes intensified, and the resulting laser light hits the target. The physician can immediately see the point that is treated and check the result.

Cryotherapy procedure

Cryotherapy is typically performed with you lying on your back. The surface of the eye is anesthetized. Your eyelids are held open with a device known as a speculum. The physician examines your retina using the indirect ophthalmoscope to see the far edge of the retina. Cryotherapy is applied with a probe connected to a cold source. The cryoprobe can be placed on the surface of the eye. When the probe is properly located, the freezing process can begin. The tip of the probe rapidly reaches a very low temperature and creates an actual freeze that extends from the soft external tissues through the wall of the eye until it reaches the retina. The physician can see the freeze directly. Multiple points of the retina can be treated in this fashion.

Vitrectomy procedure

Vitrectomy is a procedure for removal of the vitreous gel, which may be extremely cloudy or may be pulling on the retina. The vitreous is then replaced with a clear fluid similar to the fluid in the eye.

Vitrectomy is performed in a darkened operating room. It requires either a local regional anesthetic or general anesthesia. General anesthesia may be preferred if you will require a more prolonged procedure or if you are anxious and unable to tolerate being awake during surgery.

Once the anesthesia has taken effect, the surgeon makes small incisions to allow access to the wall of your eye. Typically, three very small openings are made through the wall of the eye into the vitreous cavity. One opening allows new clear fluids to flow in. This maintains the correct pressure within the eye and replaces the vitreous fluid that may be removed in the surgery. The other two openings are used by the surgeon, one to illuminate and the other to manipulate the tissues of your eye. An operating microscope is positioned over your eye, and with various contact lenses, the surgeon can see the vitreous cavity, its contents, and the underlying retinal tissue.

The initial step is to clear the vitreous cavity. In patients who have a hemorrhage, the vitreous often is partially or completely filled with blood. This blood is removed, and the cavity is filled with clear fluid. Patients who have a clear vitreous but underlying scar tissue or retinal detachment also undergo removal of the vitreous gel and replacement of it with clear fluid. This allows the surgeon to pass the required instruments safely to the retinal surface without snagging or pulling on the vitreous gel.

Once the vitreous cavity has been cleared, surgery on the surface of the retina can be done. This may include vacuuming blood from the surface. Patients often have scar tissue and blood vessels extending from the retina up into the vitreous cavity. These scars can be cut free from the retina and treated directly to seal their blood vessels. Scarring that has caused retinal detachment can be removed, and the detached retina will often gradually settle back into its normal position.

The surgeon can insert a probe through the vitreous to deliver laser treatment to the retina at the completion of the surgery. In some instances, patients will have underlying tears or holes in the retina. Often, these are managed with laser treatment combined with a gas bubble. A gas bubble holds the margins of the retinal tear against the back wall of the eye until the laser treatment can create a secure seal.

Various gases are used to hold the retina in place until healing is complete. Some gases last only a few days, and others last several months. While gas is in the eye, you will notice markedly reduced vision. As the gas is absorbed, you frequently will notice a portion of your vision is blocked by the gas bubble, but the area not covered by the gas has normal vision. The gas bubble will separate into multiple tiny bubbles and then be absorbed. As absorption takes place, the vitreous cavity is naturally refilled by the eye's normal production of aqueous fluid. After vitrectomy, with or without gas injection, the vitreous cavity is refilled by the naturally occurring aqueous fluid. Before your surgery, the aqueous filled only the small front portion of the eye, but now it fills the vitreous cavity as well. The vitreous is not replaced, and its absence is not damaging to the eye.

Once your retinopathy has been stabilized by vitrectomy, it typically remains stable for the rest of your life. It is uncommon for vitrectomy patients to have recurrent proliferation later in life. Sight-threatening complications are rare. However, it is common for cataracts to form in eyes that have had vitrectomy. You should be aware that cataract surgery may be required in an eye that has had successful vitrectomy.

What do you need to do after having treatment for retinopathy?

The most important thing you can do before and after any kind of treatment for retinopathy is to control your blood glucose and blood pressure levels.

Laser

After laser treatment, you may not need any eye medication. Some patients need a brief course of eye drops to reduce inflammation. Postoperative pain rarely needs to be treated even with oral pain relievers. If only anesthetic drops were used, you usually do not require a patch on your eye. However, if a regional anesthetic was used, the eye may be patched until the anesthesia wears off and the eye is working normally.

Cryotherapy

After treatment, the outer surface of the eye is often swollen. It may appear red for 1–2 weeks. You may have eyedrops for inflammation. You may feel a moderate degree of discomfort, depending on the amount of treatment you needed. Oral pain medications can usually make you feel better.

Vitrectomy

Vitrectomy is generally an inpatient procedure. A variety of medications may be used after surgery, including drops to dilate the pupil, inhibit infection, and reduce inflammation. Depending on the extent of the surgery, you may require pain medication immediately by injection, but more commonly, you will be comfortable using oral pain medications.

You will have swelling and redness of the tissues of the eye. The swelling and redness will go away over approximately 3 weeks. At that time, you can resume wearing contact lenses, if you wear them. You may be asked to maintain certain head positions, as you may have a small amount of hemorrhage in the eye. To help clear the hemorrhage, you will be asked to sleep with the head of the bed elevated and to avoid bending over.

If a gas bubble was used, you may be asked to position yourself to allow the gas bubble to press against treated areas of the retina until the gas is absorbed and replaced by the aqueous fluid of the eye. **You should not fly in any aircraft until the bubble is gone.** If you must have another general anesthetic during the postoperative period, be sure to tell your physician about the gas in your eye. Such anesthesia can be done safely, but the anesthesiologist must know that the gas is in the vitreous cavity of your eye. Depending on your vision in the other eye and requirements for transportation or work, you may need a period of inactivity, including a leave of absence from work.

How does vision change after treatment for retinopathy?

Patients treated for macular swelling rarely notice tiny blank spots in their field of vision, and these usually are not troublesome. After scatter treatment, some patients may notice a decrease in night vision, color vision, or peripheral vision. These symptoms may progress gradually over many years. A temporary decrease in central vision is common, and some patients may experience a permanent slight reduction in vision. Temporary glare and difficulty focusing on near objects is a common occurrence after scatter treatment but generally goes away after one day to several weeks.

It is not possible to predict how your vision will be improved after laser treatment or vitrectomy. There are many causes for loss of vision, and you may have several of them. For instance, treating macular swelling or abnormal blood vessels will not alter the age-related development of cataracts. Removal of hemorrhage by vitrectomy will clear the path for light to reach the retina, but the health of the underlying retina can't be determined until surgery is done.

The fear that laser or surgery may harm vision often makes a patient decide to delay therapy. Although there are potential risks in any form of treatment, the benefits of treating retinopathy greatly outweigh the risk of treatment. If you don't get treatment, diabetic retinopathy is usually progressive and sight threatening. Treatment with laser and vitrectomy have been proven to benefit vision greatly. The best time for laser surgery is before you lose any vision. Detecting retinopathy just as it reaches a treatable stage is the most important factor in preventing visual loss.

How effective are these treatments for retinopathy?

Four nationwide clinical trials showed that scatter laser surgery for proliferative retinopathy and local laser surgery for macular edema significantly reduce your risk of vision loss. A person with proliferative retinopathy who does not get treatment may have a 60% risk of severe vision loss over 5 years. Laser surgery reduces this risk to less than 2%.

What else can you do to prevent or control retinopathy?

People with type 1 and type 2 diabetes who control their blood glucose significantly reduce their risk of any retinopathy or slow the progression of retinopathy once it is present, and reduce the need for laser surgery. You would be wise to try to keep your blood glucose close to the targets set for you.

Does diabetes cause blurred or fluctuating vision?

Uncontrolled blood glucose levels can blur your vision. Frequently, higher levels of blood glucose can cause you to become more near-sighted. Your distance vision may become blurred, while near vision may actually seem clearer. Some people may even find they don't need reading glasses. Such changes in vision may be temporary.

What are cataracts?

A cataract is any cloudiness in the lens of the eye. Cataracts tend to develop at a younger age and progress more rapidly in people with diabetes. Cataracts generally affect people 60 years of age or older, and most cataracts progress gradually. It is not unusual, however, for people with diabetes to develop cataracts in their 30s or 40s, and the progression of the cataract can be dramatic. Cataracts specifically related to diabetes are sometimes caused by very poorly controlled blood glucose levels.

What are the symptoms of cataracts?

Symptoms of cataracts may include a dimming of vision, decreased reading vision, higher reading light requirements, or difficulty driving. Sometimes, cataracts cause car headlights to have a star-burst or sparkler effect.

What is the treatment for cataracts?

When cataracts interfere enough with vision to prevent you from performing necessary tasks of daily living, surgery may be indicated. Cataract surgery today is generally performed as an outpatient procedure. In most cases, the lens is surgically removed from the eye. A plastic lens is then implanted in the eye. Generally, the surgeon will intentionally leave the lens capsule in place in the eye. This capsule continues to separate the two sections of the eye.

Cataract surgery itself is not performed with a laser; however, with time, the lens capsule may become cloudy, much like an original cataract. This condition is frequently referred to as an aftercataract. Aftercataracts are routinely treated with a laser, which opens a permanent clear hole in the cloudy lens capsule. The laser used for this treatment is different from the lasers used to treat diabetic retinopathy.

After cataract surgery, glasses are usually still required for best vision—for reading, for distance, or for both. The lens implant fixes the focus of the eye for only one distance, but glasses allow the flexibility of focusing at different distances.

What is glaucoma?

As a person with diabetes, you are twice as likely to develop glaucoma as someone without diabetes. Glaucoma is a condition in which the pressure inside the eye causes damage to the optic nerve. Generally, increased pressure causes damage. The eye constantly produces and drains a fluid known as the aqueous. This fluid is not a component of our tears and does not come to the outer surface of the eye. The balance of production and drainage determines the pressure in the eye (see Figure 4-1).

The same loss of blood supply that causes new blood vessels to grow on the retina also causes them to grow across the drainage network and block the fluid from leaving the eye. The eye keeps on making fluid but cannot drain it. The eye is rigid; it does not enlarge. Therefore, the pressure inside the eye increases and eventually damages the optic nerve.

There are many types of glaucoma. The most common form of glaucoma is open-angle glaucoma. It is caused by a reduction in the outflow of aqueous in the drainage network, which is also called the filtration angle. Usually, open-angle glaucoma causes no symptoms or changes in vision until damage is advanced. Damage usually occurs over a prolonged period and progresses gradually.

In angle-closure glaucoma, fluid can't drain because the filtration angle is too narrow. Angle closure can occur spontaneously or can even be caused by dilation of the pupils, which is a normal part of a comprehensive eye examination. A comprehensive eye examination, however, can usually determine whether an eye is prone to angle closure, and treatment can prevent angle-closure attacks. A person with angle-closure glaucoma may experience excruciating pain in the eye and rapid decrease in vision, although pain may be caused by other problems such as foreign bodies in the eye or scratches on the cornea. If angle closure is not complete, a person may have angle-closure attacks, which may result in the appearance of haloes around lights. Diabetes does not pose a greater risk for angle-closure glaucoma.

Another type of glaucoma is neovascular glaucoma. In neovascular glaucoma, new blood vessels grow on the surface of the iris and eventually reach and block the filtration angle. Diabetes can be a risk factor for neovascular glaucoma, particularly if proliferative diabetic retinopathy is present. There may be no symptoms, or there may be symptoms similar to those of angle-closure glaucoma.

What is the treatment for glaucoma?

Treatment for glaucoma depends on the type of glaucoma. Open-angle glaucoma is initially treated with eyedrops. Laser treatments to the filtration angle are sometimes indicated if the glaucoma does not respond to eyedrops or other medications.

Laser treatments can be used to create a small hole in the iris of the eye, allowing fluid to pass from one section of the eye to the other. Such treatment, called a laser iridotomy, usually cures and prevents angle-closure glaucoma, although careful follow-up evaluations are needed. Angle-closure glaucoma is an emergency and may be treated with eyedrops, laser therapy, and/or surgery.

Neovascular glaucoma is usually treated with laser surgery to the retina, because the new vessels grow as the result of retinal dysfunction. Eyedrops or laser treatment to the vessels themselves may be necessary if the glaucoma does not respond to laser treatment of the retina. Once again, it is crucial to have follow-up visits to the eye-care specialist during the active stages of these conditions.

Can diabetes affect the optic nerve in other ways?

Diabetes can damage blood vessels and restrict blood flow through them. The optic nerve is damaged whenever it does not receive adequate blood supply. Initially, it swells. It may then recover, but some atrophy often follows. The atrophy, which consists of a loss of nerve fibers, is permanent and may result in loss of a portion of your field of vision or both the peripheral and central vision.

A loss of blood supply to the visual nerve pathways in the brain can also damage your vision. This loss of circulation is commonly called a stroke (chapter 7). Sometimes a clot may block a blood vessel briefly and then move on. This will cause a temporary loss of some part or all of your vision that clears up on its own. Bring these symptoms to the attention of your doctor to determine the cause and location of the obstruction and to prevent it from happening again.

What happens when you have double vision?

Diabetes can sometimes result in double vision. The position of the human eye is controlled by six muscles that surround the eye. Each eye has its own muscles and nerve supply, and the movements of both eyes are coordinated so that they maintain focus simultaneously on a given visual target. Diabetes can do damage to both blood vessels and nerves. If one nerve is impaired by lack of blood supply, the muscle cannot move the eye, and the coordination is disrupted. The two eyes are focused on two different targets, and the brain gets two distinct images, causing double vision.

Decreased blood supply to the nerves that activate the muscles of the eye can cause a full or partial paralysis of the eye muscles supplied by the nerve. This is called mononeuropathy. Symptoms of mononeuropathy can include sudden onset of double vision, drooping of the eyelid, and sometimes pain over the affected eye. Treatment of this condition can be to patch either eye to eliminate one of the two images or to use an optical device called a prism in a spectacle lens in an attempt to align the two eyes. In general, the nerve regains its function over several months, and the eyes again track together. Rarely, surgery on the muscle is required to realign the eyes so they can maintain a single image.

Double vision may be the first sign of serious or life-threatening conditions. Immediate eye examination and careful evaluation by a doctor familiar with diabetic eye disease is critical.

Does physical activity affect retinopathy?

In general, physical activity and exercise do not affect vision in cases of macular edema or nonproliferative retinopathy. In cases of active proliferative retinopathy, however—particularly if vitreous hemorrhage, fibrous tissue, or significant new vessel growth is present—some types of physical activity might cause those new blood vessels to rupture, resulting in vitreous hemorrhage. Also, exertion may lead to retinal detachment if significant retinal traction is present. Contact sports that involve jarring, high-impact aerobics, and lifting free weights might cause you problems. Your comprehensive eye examination will help you and your physician determine the best level of exercise.

What can you do to reduce your risk of vision loss?

Take an active role in your own eye care. The best way to prevent severe diabetic retinopathy is to control your blood glucose and blood pressure levels. You should also

- have regular eye examinations as your eye doctor recommends (Table 4-1)
- maintain good control of other medical conditions, especially kidney disease, high blood pressure, and high cholesterol and triglycerides

Table 4-1. Suggested Frequency of Eye Examinations

Type of Diabetes	Recommended 1st Examination	Routine Minimal Follow-Up
Type 1	For people 10 yrs or older 3–5 years after onset	Yearly
Type 2	On diagnosis	Yearly
During Pregnancy	• Before conception for counseling • Early in 1st trimester	• Each trimester • More frequently as indicated • 3–6 months postpartum

More frequent examinations may be necessary based on the level of retinopathy and the presence of other medical conditions.

In conclusion

With regular and lifelong eye examinations, more than 98% of severe vision loss from diabetic retinopathy can be prevented.

This chapter was written by M. Gilbert Grand, MD; Lloyd Paul Aiello, MD, PhD; Jerry D. Cavallerano, OD, PhD; and Mami A. Iwamoto, MD.

5

Heart Disease

Introduction

Adults with diabetes are three times more likely to die of cardiovascular disease than the general population. Diabetes puts you at serious risk for several forms of heart and vascular disease—coronary artery disease, heart attack, and sudden death. Keeping your blood sugar as close to normal as possible can lower your risk of cardiovascular problems.

What is coronary artery disease?

Coronary artery disease (CAD) is an illness in which some of your heart muscle does not receive enough blood, oxygen, and nutrients because the blood vessels which supply the heart are partially or completely blocked. The most common cause of CAD is atherosclerosis, or hardening of the arteries. In this disease, cholesterol builds up in the walls of the blood vessels gradually over many years. The process is complex. There is usually some initial damage to the lining of the major arteries of the heart. Common causes of injury include high blood pressure, diabetes, smoking, and high blood cholesterol levels. The body's response to this injury encourages scavenger cells (macrophages) to enter the damaged areas to repair the injury. However, macrophages, and substances they produce, contribute to blocking the vessels. After many cycles of injury and attempted repair, deposits of cholesterol and scar tissue build up and block the vessel.

What puts you at risk for developing CAD?

Your risk factors for CAD are diabetes, a family history of CAD, high blood pressure, smoking, high cholesterol, aging, sedentary lifestyle, high triglycerides, and obesity.

People with pre-diabetes or impaired glucose tolerance (IGT) are at higher risk for developing angina and heart attack, and people with diabetes are at an even higher risk. How long you have had diabetes also increases the chances of developing CAD. If you have had diabetes for 15–20 years, you are 10 times as likely to develop CAD as people in the general population.

Years of cigarette smoking increase your risk, too. The good news is that quitting helps. The risk level decreases when you have not smoked for 5 years.

The higher your blood cholesterol level, the higher your risk. There is a direct relationship between LDL (bad) cholesterol and CAD—risk increases as your LDL level increases. However, raising your levels of HDL (good) cholesterol protects you against CAD (chapter 6).

What are the symptoms of CAD?

When 50–75% of a blood vessel is blocked, the limited blood flow can cause symptoms. Generally, the symptoms occur first with exercise, because the heart requires more fuel when heart rate and blood pressure increase. The most common symptom is pain (angina) or pressure in the chest (Table 5-1). However, the symptoms can vary. The pain usually comes on gradually over several minutes. It may become more severe, or remain mild and then go away. The pain may move to the left arm, shoulder, armpit, or left side of the neck or jaw. Typically, it

Table 5-1. Symptoms of Coronary Artery Disease

- Chest pain/pressure
  - Under the breast bone, in the left arm, shoulder, neck, or jaw
  - Pressure (or tightness)
  - Gradual onset (over 30 seconds to minutes)
  - Gradually goes away
  - Related to physical or emotional stress
- Shortness of breath
  - Usually associated with chest pain or physical or emotional stress
- Nausea
  - Usually associated with chest pain or shortness of breath and physical or emotional stress
- Palpitation, Fainting, Sudden death
  - Related to irregular heartbeat caused by insufficient blood flow to the heart muscle

comes on with exercise and is relieved by rest. However, the pain can come on at rest, or even awaken you from sleep. The pain may also begin during emotional stress, such as during an argument.

Some people complain of nausea or discomfort in the upper abdomen, often mistaking it for heartburn. Sometimes these symptoms are relieved by belching or by taking antacids, which can be confusing for both you and your physician. These are also symptoms of gastroparesis, gallbladder disease, and other gastrointestinal problems that people with diabetes are more likely to have (chapter 13). Also, some people with diabetes have nerve damage and cannot feel the heart pain, just as some people develop foot ulcers in part because they can't feel injuries to their feet (chapters 3 and 11). Your only symptoms may be caused by the part of the heart muscle that is not receiving enough blood. You may be short of breath because your heart cannot pump blood out into the body, so the blood backs up into the lungs. Sometimes patients become weak because the brain is not getting the blood and oxygen it needs. A heart that is receiving insufficient blood may beat rapidly or irregularly.

When symptoms last only 2–15 minutes and do not occur more frequently or at lower levels of exercise, and heart tests show no evidence of permanent damage, you have *stable angina*. When the symptoms abruptly get worse or begin occurring at rest, the pattern is called *unstable angina*, a warning sign of serious heart trouble. These symptoms may precede a heart attack.

How does neuropathy affect your cardiovascular system?

Autonomic nerves control your heart rate and blood pressure. Normally, blood pressure and heart rate change slightly throughout the day in response to lying, sitting, and standing; stress; exercise; breathing patterns; and sleep. If the nerves to the heart and blood vessels are damaged by diabetes, your blood pressure and heart rate may respond more slowly to these factors.

If the nerves that regulate blood pressure are damaged, blood pressure can drop quickly when you stand up and not return to a normal level as quickly as it should. You can feel lightheaded and dizzy, see black spots, or even pass out. This is called *orthostatic hypotension* (chapter 12).

If nerves that control heart rate are damaged, the heart rate tends to be fast and does not change as quickly in response to breathing patterns, exercise, stress, or sleep. This is diagnosed by measuring the rise and fall of heart rate as you breathe deeply or by a Valsalva maneuver (when you bear down as hard as you can). This serious complication may increase your risk for an irregular heartbeat.

Autonomic neuropathy can keep you from feeling chest pain, so you may have a "silent" heart attack, which is a heart attack without pain. Sudden high blood sugar levels may be your symptom of a heart attack (chapter 12).

How can your doctor diagnose CAD?

Usually, the symptoms alert you and your health care provider to the possibility that you have it. The more classic your symptoms (location, character, relationship to exercise, etc.) and the greater your number of risk factors, the more likely it is that you have CAD. At this point, any of several diagnostic tests can help confirm the diagnosis.

An ECG performed at rest can help the physician diagnose a heart attack that occurred sometime in the past (or one that is occurring at the time of the ECG). As many as one-third of all heart attacks are clinically silent—that is, you don't notice any symptoms at the time of the heart attack—but an ECG performed at a later date indicates what happened. However, coronary blockages that have not yet caused a heart attack may not show up on a resting ECG.

Stress testing is performed by examining you and obtaining ECGs before, during, and after you exercise on a treadmill or exercise bicycle. The level of exercise is increased in steps until you develop symptoms that cause you to stop, you become tired, the ECG becomes very abnormal, or you reach a maximum target heart rate. Stress testing can be performed with an ECG, a cardiac ultrasound test, or a radioactive scan to determine whether you have blood flow problems. Ultrasound and radioactive tracers are monitored with the ECG. When you have partially or completely blocked coronary arteries and you exercise, some of the heart muscle may not receive enough blood. It moves differently, and this shows up on the ECG. The stress ECG is only moderately accurate for diagnosing CAD. It gives false positives. Only about 70% of patients with a positive test will actually have obstructions in their coronary arteries. That's why most people have both exercise stress testing and a heart imaging test with ultrasound or radioactive scan.

An echocardiogram (heart ultrasound) or nuclear imaging done before and immediately after exercise give more accurate information. Both tests help to determine the level of blood flow to different parts of the heart, so the doctor can see how many and how large the obstructions are. The echo and nuclear stress tests detect abnormal coronary arteries in about 90% of people tested. But only 90% of these people actually have significant obstructions. The more severe the CAD is, the more likely the tests will show it.

What if you cannot exercise?

Many people with suspected CAD cannot exercise because they have another disease such as asthma, emphysema, peripheral vascular disease with claudication (aching in the legs during exercise), or amputation. For these people, cardiologists use chemical stress tests. In these tests, the echocardiogram or nuclear imaging is done before and after stress with drugs such as dobutamine (which increases the work of the heart), or adenosine or dipyridamole (which expand the arteries of the heart). The accuracy of stress testing using drugs is similar to that of tests using exercise.

What happens when your test is positive?

If your stress test is positive, your doctor may start you on oral medications to reduce your symptoms, slow the progression of CAD, and extend your life. Or you may be scheduled for *cardiac catheterization* and *angiography*. In this procedure, the cardiologist examines your heart using a plastic catheter (tube) inserted into an artery (usually in the groin) after you've been given a local anesthetic. The catheters are threaded up the major vessels into the chest so that blood pressures can be checked in the different chambers of the heart.

X-ray dye can flow through the tubes into your heart and heart arteries so that the physician can observe the overall function of your heart, whether some walls are moving normally, and whether there are large obstructions in the arteries. Depending on the results, you may not need special treatment. Your stress test gave a false positive result. Otherwise, you may need oral or topical medicines for angina, a procedure to open the artery mechanically (*angioplasty*) or bypass surgery. These decisions are complex and depend on your anatomy, the number and severity of blockages, their locations, the size of the openings in the vessels, and the pump function of your heart.

What medications should you take for CAD?

Generally, nitroglycerine or beta blockers are given for CAD.

Nitroglycerin

Several classes of medication are available if your physician chooses this therapy (Table 5-2). One of the oldest is nitroglycerin or similar medications. These medications can be taken orally, under the tongue, or by patch or ointment on the skin. They reduce or prevent angina (chest pain) by lowering the blood pressure and filling pressure of the heart and by dilating (expanding) the heart arteries and helping balance oxygen supply and demand. These medications can only be used for 12–14 hours per day because the body does not respond to them if they are used continuously. They can cause headaches and light-headedness. There is no evidence that these medications prolong life.

Beta blockers

The beta blockers (propranolol [Inderal]), atenolol [Tenormin], metoprolol [Lopressor], etc.) are another group of medications used to treat angina. These drugs reduce your symptoms by lowering the heart rate and blood pressure and by partially blocking the effects of epinephrine on the heart. In addition to

Table 5-2. Treatments for Stable Coronary Artery Disease

- **Medical therapy**
  - Nitrates
  - Beta blockers
  - Calcium-channel blockers (not recommended)
  - Cholesterol-lowering medication
  - Aspirin
- **Catheter-based therapy**
  - Balloon angioplasty
  - Atherectomy (rotablator)
  - Directional atherectomy
- **Coronary artery bypass**

reducing symptoms of CAD, they help prevent irregular heartbeats. For people who have had heart attacks, these drugs dramatically prolong life over the 3–5 years after the heart attack. Beta blockers may also prolong life in some people with congestive heart failure.

Beta blockers can give some people problems. People with type 1 diabetes who are prone to low blood glucose need to check more often because beta blockers can dull the body's warning signs of low blood glucose. People with type 1 and type 2 diabetes may find that beta blockers upset their blood glucose control. The drugs may raise serum triglycerides while lowering HDL (good) cholesterol. They may make peripheral vascular disease worse. People with asthma or other forms of lung disease associated with wheezing may not be able to tolerate these drugs because they can make wheezing worse. Beta blockers may also slow the heart rate too much in patients who already have a low heart rate.

Calcium-channel blockers

The third major class of drugs for angina are the calcium-channel blockers (nifedipine [Procardia], verapamil [Calan], diltiazem [Cardizem], amlodipine [Norvasc], etc.). These drugs treat angina by reducing blood pressure and dilating the coronary arteries. Some of these drugs also reduce heart rate. However, people with diabetes are advised not to use them because of serious side effects.

What else can you do?

Take control of the ABCs of diabetes. A is for the A1C test—a measure of your average blood glucose control. The suggested target is below 7. Have an A1C test at least twice a year. B is for blood pressure. High blood pressure makes your heart work too hard. The target is below 130/80. Have your blood pressure checked at every doctor's visit. C is for cholesterol. LDL "bad" cholesterol builds up and clogs your arteries. The suggested target is below 100. Have it checked at least once a year. Actions you can take to protect your heart are listed in Table 5-3.

If your doctor finds cholesterol plaque (buildup), especially in the coronary blood vessels, your cholesterol levels are too high. You can control cholesterol levels with careful attention to diet, weight control, and exercise. You may need drugs, such as a statin, too (chapter 6).

To further reduce your risk of heart disease lose weight and stop smoking. Strong studies suggest that long-term treatment with aspirin helps prevent heart attacks. There is also some evidence that eating foods containing antioxidants (vitamins A, C, and E) may help prevent or delay the development of CAD. This is a great reason to add more vegetables and fruits to your daily meals. Try vegetables with deep colors, such as carrots, sweet potatoes, tomatoes, spinach, broccoli, cantaloupe, pumpkin, apricots, and citrus fruits. The main food

Table 5-3. Actions to Take for Good Heart Health

Get physical activity every day.

Eat less fat and salt.

Eat more fiber. Choose whole grains, fruits,
vegetables, and beans.

Stay at a healthy weight.

Stop smoking. Ask your provider for help.

Take medicines as prescribed, especially blood
pressure and cholesterol-lowering medications.

Ask your doctor about taking aspirin.

sources of vitamin E are vegetable oils, green and leafy vegetables, wheat germ (refrigerate because it spoils quickly), whole-grain products, nuts, and seeds.

Will you need angioplasty or bypass surgery?

If you and your physician decide that your coronary arteries need surgical repair or bypass of blockages, several options are available. There are procedures to open the artery mechanically (angioplasty) or to bypass the obstruction in the blood vessel and get the blood flowing again. Studies show that a bypass yields better results for people with diabetes.

Angioplasty

A balloon attached to a catheter is inserted into the narrowed artery and inflated to open it. The balloon is inflated many times during the angioplasty to increase the likelihood of the artery staying open. When the balloon is expanded, the cholesterol deposit is reshaped and there is usually a small, controlled tear in the lining of the blood vessel.

A stent is a small device, usually made of metal in the shape of a spring or mesh cylinder, that may be positioned in the coronary artery at the site of the obstruction. It is compressed until the balloon inflates it to hold the vessel open and prevent the cholesterol deposit from blocking the artery again.

Some blood vessels cannot be dilated with a balloon with or without a stent. These blockages may be opened with a *rotablator*, which has a motorized burr (much like a dentist's drill) located at the tip of the catheter. Some devices actually remove some of the cholesterol plaque. Stents are frequently used in this procedure, too.

Recent data suggests that an angioplasty may not be the best choice for people with diabetes. There are serious complications. In some cases, the coronary vessel will re-close abruptly because of clotting at the site of the dilation or tearing of the vessel. Nearly all patients who have angioplasty, with or without stents, receive drugs to prevent clotting. A stent appears to reduce the likelihood of the vessel closing abruptly. Without stents, as many as one-third of the vessels that are opened may renarrow over 3–9 months. However, even when stents have been used, the blood vessels of people with diabetes are more likely to renarrow after angioplasty.

Bypass surgery

Coronary artery bypass surgery is often chosen because it is effective for patients with extensive CAD and those with less serious disease but depressed heart pump function. **Studies have shown that bypass is much more successful than angioplasty in people with diabetes over time.** During bypass surgery, an artery taken from the inside of the chest wall or veins removed from the leg are used to bypass the narrowed portion of the vessel and to deliver blood beyond the blockage. This procedure relieves symptoms of angina, may help damaged heart muscle to improve its pumping ability, and, in some patients, prevent heart attack and prolong life.

The veins used for bypass grafting are usually removed from the lower portion of one or both legs, depending on how many bypasses are necessary. The surgical procedure may require 4–6 hours, or even longer if it is a repeat procedure or if a heart valve must be repaired or replaced at the same time. Complications of bypass surgery include heart attack, bleeding, infection of the breast bone (sternum), or infection of the site from which the veins are taken. Complications are more frequent in people with diabetes, especially infection and difficulties with healing. However, most people with diabetes have coronary artery bypass surgery with excellent results.

What is a heart attack?

A heart attack occurs when a coronary artery is clogged or blocked suddenly. Before the heart attack occurs, there may be a gradual blockage of a coronary vessel with cholesterol plaque, as we discussed earlier. The difference between stable CAD and a heart attack is that during the heart attack, one of the cholesterol plaques has cracked, causing a hemorrhage that blocks the vessel, or the vessel has narrowed until a tiny clot or clump of platelets can block it and deprive the muscle downstream of the blood necessary for survival. Sometimes, some of the cells that line the coronary artery are sheared off by a rapid blood flow or some other damaging process. The tissue that is exposed promotes vigorous clotting that can block the vessel suddenly. Sometimes blood flows into the exposed cholesterol plaque and shears off a portion of it, forming a flap valve that suddenly blocks the vessel. However the blockage occurs, it prevents blood from reaching some of the heart muscle, causing part of that muscle to die.

What are the symptoms of a heart attack?

Classically, a heart attack presents with a sudden onset of severe, crushing chest pain located under the sternum (breast bone) and spreading to the left armpit, arm, shoulder, neck, and jaw (Table 5-4). If pain is rated on a 1–10 scale, with 1 being very mild and 10 being the worst pain ever experienced, heart attack pain is often 8–10. At the beginning, the pain may be less severe and may come and go over a period of hours, but severe pain is common. The pain can be associated with nausea, vomiting, sweating, palpitations, and shortness of breath.

Sometimes people will have only abdominal discomfort or back pain. Women may have symptoms different from those in men. If a heart attack is suspected, you (or your family) should call an ambulance to take you to the nearest hospital. Speedy transport to the hospital is critical because 50% of all people who die of heart attack do so within the first hour. Many of these early deaths are preventable with prompt medical attention. The earlier treatment is given, the more heart muscle can be saved.

People with diabetes often have different or no symptoms of heart attack. Silent heart attacks are common. If you have

Table 5-4. Symptoms of Heart Attack

- Crushing chest pain
  - Left anterior chest
  - Movement to left shoulder, neck, jaw
  - Bandlike pain/tightness
  - Persistent, more than 15 minutes
- Shortness of breath
- Nausea/vomiting
- Sweating
- Palpitations
  - Fainting
  - Near fainting

several risk factors for heart disease, be alert for any heart attack symptoms, including sudden out-of-control blood glucose levels. It is not unusual for people with diabetes to have the symptoms of nausea and shortness of breath but no chest pain because of damage to the sensory nerves of the heart. Discuss with your doctor whether you need any tests. Heart attack is common in people with diabetes—30–50% more common than in other people of similar age, sex, and risk factors. The risk of having another heart attack is increased, and the risk is higher for people with type 1 than for those with type 2 diabetes.

How is a heart attack diagnosed?

A heart attack can be diagnosed with an ECG. It can also be detected by blood tests, because with injury to the heart muscle, certain proteins from the damaged heart leak into the blood. Some of these proteins are unique to the heart and provide an extremely accurate diagnosis. The level of these proteins in the blood indicates the magnitude of the heart injury. During hospitalization for heart attack, you may have a cardiac catheterization performed to determine whether angioplasty or bypass surgery is appropriate. You may have an echocardiogram and a stress test to evaluate overall heart pump function and to assess your risk for more heart attacks after you are discharged. If you have poor pump function and/or imbalance between oxygen supply and demand of the heart, you are at substantially increased risk for another heart attack.

What is the treatment for heart attack?

The first treatment is to interrupt the process of the heart attack and to get blood flowing to save some of the heart muscle that would otherwise die (Table 5-5). The sooner blood flow is reestablished, the more heart muscle is saved, and the fewer long-term complications there will be. You may be given

Table 5-5. Treatment for Heart Attack

Initial
• **Thrombolysis (clot dissolver)**
• **Immediate angioplasty**
• **Aspirin**
• **Beta blockers**
Long term
• **Beta blockers**
• **Angiotensin-converting enzyme inhibitors**
• **Cholesterol reduction**
• **Aspirin**
• **Risk factor modification**
— **Smoking cessation**
— **Hypertension management**
— **Diabetes management**
— **Exercise**

clot-dissolving medications administered intravenously (through a vein), such as tissue plasminogen activator (TPA) or streptokinase, or you may have an immediate angioplasty.

The decision of whether to use medication or angioplasty is often determined by technical factors, such as the availability of a catheterization laboratory and whether you have conditions that clot-dissolving medications would make worse, such as a recent stroke, bleeding, or surgery (including retinal laser treatment).

If clot-dissolving medications are given within 1 hour of the onset of symptoms, mortality rates can be cut in half. This therapy opens clotted vessels equally well in all patients regardless of whether they have diabetes. Likewise, the complications of thrombolytic therapy, including bleeding and stroke, are the same for all patients. After the clot dissolves, some people have follow-up angiography and angioplasty. This is not recommended for people with diabetes, because this approach puts you at three times the risk of complications, including death.

Several follow-up therapies have been studied extensively. The use of beta blockers prolongs life after heart attack in all patients. Drugs that prevent progressive cardiac enlargement and lower blood pressure (angiotensin-converting enzyme inhibitors, or ACE inhibitors) successfully lower the risk of death over the first 3–5 years after a heart attack for all patients, regardless of diabetes. Long-term therapy routinely includes aspirin, lowering cholesterol, and smoking cessation.

What is congestive heart failure?

Congestive heart failure (CHF) is a condition in which the heart is unable to pump sufficient blood to meet the needs of the body, particularly kidney function. When this occurs, the body retains water. Symptoms are shortness of breath, decreased ability to exercise, and swelling of the feet and ankles. CHF is a common illness, with 400,000 new diagnoses each year in the U.S. and nearly 3 million people in the U.S. who currently have it. CHF is even more common in the elderly, doubling with each decade over the age of 45 years. It is the leading and most expensive cause of hospitalization in patients over the age of 65 years.

How are diabetes and CHF connected?

If you have diabetes, you have an increased chance of developing CHF because of other cardiovascular problems linked with diabetes, including CAD, heart attack, and hypertension, all of which can cause CHF. However, in the Framingham study, which has followed the heart status of patients over many years, even after all patients with CAD and rheumatic heart disease (heart valve disease) were excluded, the risk of developing CHF was increased four to five times in patients with diabetes. The increased risk was still observed after the effects of age, blood pressure, and cholesterol levels were taken into account.

It appears that diabetes has negative effects on both contraction and relaxation of the heart beyond any difficulties caused by CAD or hypertension. The small vessels of the heart may be affected by diabetes, just as the small vessels in the kidney, the eye, and other organs are affected. Studies of the hearts of diabetic patients who have died have shown a thickening of the walls of the small vessels of the heart and scarring around these vessels as well. Studies of the blood flow of the heart using advanced nuclear imaging techniques have shown that the small vessels of the heart cannot dilate well even in response to powerful drugs. These studies suggest that the small vessels of the heart are abnormal in anatomy and function.

Diabetes affects both the pumping and filling properties of the heart. The heart's inability to pump blood forward makes you feel fatigued even before you exercise. If your heart can't relax, it is difficult for it to fill during the resting phase of a cardiac cycle. This is reflected by high pressures in the heart, which lead to increased blood filling the lungs (backup of fluid). This process makes it difficult for you to breathe, particularly when lying down but also during exercise. The body's attempts to compensate can lead to further fluid accumulation, ankle and leg swelling, and racing and irregular heart rhythms.

How is CHF diagnosed?

The diagnosis of CHF depends on your history of shortness of breath, reduced ability to exercise, and swollen feet and ankles (Table 5-6). The diagnosis is usually confirmed with a chest X ray and an echocardiogram. The echocardiogram allows the

Table 5-6. Symptoms of Congestive Heart Failure

- Shortness of breath
  — With exercise
  — When reclining
- Awakening from sleep
  — For shortness of breath
  — To urinate
- Easy fatiguability
- Swelling of the feet, ankles, and legs
- Palpitations

cardiologist to distinguish between poor forward heart pump function and increased heart stiffness or poor relaxation—patients often have both. The distinction is important because the treatment for poor forward pump function may be different from the treatment for problems with relaxation.

The most common problem is poor forward pump function. This is usually treated with a combination of medications, including digoxin to increase the force of the heart's contraction, diuretics to help remove excess fluid from the body, and ACE inhibitors. ACE inhibitors help patients with heart failure by blocking the production of a hormone (angiotensin II) that causes some arteries to constrict. The body constricts these arteries to direct the blood flow to organs that need it most (brain, heart, kidney). Unfortunately, the body's response is excessive and increases the work the heart must perform at a time when it is failing and cannot handle the extra work. Treatment with ACE inhibitors relaxes some of these arteries, allowing the heart to work more effectively. Treatment of CHF with drugs of this class (enalapril [Vasotec], captopril

[Capoten], ramipril [Altace], etc.) reduces symptoms, hospitalizations, and mortality in a wide range of patients.

Will the treatment of heart problems change in the future?

There are frequent advances in management of heart disease spanning every aspect of cardiovascular disease, diagnosis, and treatment. These improvements apply equally to all patients regardless of whether they have diabetes. New stress testing procedures are being developed to improve the accuracy of the diagnosis of CAD so that fewer patients need cardiac catheterization and coronary angiography.

New devices are being introduced almost monthly to improve on angioplasty and stent procedures. In addition, new oral medications are being introduced for the treatment of angina and high blood pressure. Heart failure management is changing rapidly with the introduction of beta-blocker therapy and other new hormone-blocking agents that seem promising. The pace of change in the diagnosis and management of heart disease is rapid and has already improved short- and long-term outcomes.

This chapter was written by Edward M. Geltman, MD.

6

Cholesterol and Other Blood Fats

What is cholesterol?

Cholesterol and other blood fats are molecules called lipids. Blood fats include triglycerides, and they actually form the fatty tissue in the human body. Fats do not mix well with water, and they have to be packaged with water-soluble proteins to form lipoproteins, so they can be transported in the blood. Cholesterol and fats have several important functions:

- to form insulation around nerves
- to make bile, which is necessary for absorbing fat and fat-soluble vitamins
- to serve as an important source of energy

The cholesterol that the body needs is made mostly in the liver. The rest comes from what you eat.

What are saturated fats?

These are fats that are hard at room temperature and are found in animal products such as beef, veal, lamb, pork, butter, cream, and whole milk. They are also found in shortening, coconut oil, and palm oil. If you eat too much of these substances, they are stored as fat and also increase the production of cholesterol in your body.

What are polyunsaturated and monounsaturated fats?

These are oils that are liquid at room temperature. The oils that contain polyunsaturated fats include sunflower, soybean, and corn. Monounsaturated fats are in canola and olive oils, nuts, and seeds, and they actually lower cholesterol. However, even these so-called good oils cause weight gain when you eat too much of them.

What are the different types of cholesterol?

Cholesterol is packaged into lipoproteins to be transported in the blood. Based on the way the cholesterol and protein are packed together and the amount of cholesterol that the lipoproteins contain, they can be classified into different kinds—high-density lipoprotein (HDL), low-density lipoprotein (LDL), and triglycerides.

What are high-density lipoproteins, or HDL?

These fats are made in the liver and intestine and contain very little cholesterol. They collect excess cholesterol from the blood and blood vessels and transport it back to the liver, where it is broken down. HDL is sometimes called the "good" cholesterol. The higher your HDL level, the better. The American Diabetes Association (ADA) recommends that you aim for an HDL level greater than 45 mg/dl for men and 55 mg/dl for women.

What are low-density lipoproteins, or LDL?

These lipoproteins contain a very high concentration of cholesterol and carry it from the liver throughout the body. This form of cholesterol is also the culprit responsible for the buildup in the walls of the arteries that leads to atherosclerosis. Some people call it the "bad" cholesterol. The higher the concentration of this form of cholesterol in the blood, the greater the chance of getting heart disease (CHD). A desirable level of LDL depends on whether you already have CHD and whether you have other risk factors that would predispose you to developing CHD. LDL levels should be below 100 mg/dl.

What are triglycerides?

These are a form of fat that is carried in the blood but is mostly stored in fat tissue. The ADA goal is a level less than 150 mg/dl. Some people think that high triglycerides are an important risk factor for CHD in women. Very high levels (greater than 1,000 mg/dl) are dangerous and can cause pancreatitis (inflammation of the pancreas).

How can I tell whether I have high cholesterol?

Unfortunately, in the early stages, it is a silent disease, much like high blood pressure. You often find out about high cholesterol when you start having chest pain or, worse still, after a heart attack. Rarely, with some hereditary forms of high cholesterol, people develop "bumps" on the skin and tendons at the elbow and ankle, and a physician might notice these during a physical exam. Have your blood tested to measure your cholesterol at regular intervals.

When should I be tested for high cholesterol?

Cholesterol testing is recommended for all individuals over the age of 20 every 2 years if they have desirable cholesterol levels. This test is called a lipoprotein profile and requires you to fast beforehand. Fasting means you may not have anything to eat or drink except for water, black coffee, or tea without milk, cream, or sugar for 9–12 hours before the test, which should be done first thing in the morning.

What makes cholesterol high or low?

The factors that can affect your cholesterol levels are heredity, age, gender, diet, weight, exercise level, alcohol intake, cigarette smoking, hypertension, and diabetes.

Heredity

Your genes can influence your cholesterol levels. If your parents have high cholesterol levels, you probably will, too.

Age and gender

Cholesterol levels increase with age. Women are protected by estrogen until menopause, but women with diabetes don't have this protection. Men older than 45, women older than 55, or postmenopausal women at any age should consider themselves at higher risk for CHD, especially if they have diabetes.

Diet

Foods high in cholesterol and saturated fat raise your LDL levels. In fact, it is believed that eating high-fat foods is the reason for the high incidence of CHD in the U.S.

Weight and exercise

Excess weight, which is usually in the form of fat, increases LDL levels. Losing weight not only decreases your LDL and triglyceride levels, it increases your HDL levels. You can get the same benefits from regular physical activity.

Alcohol

Small quantities of alcohol can raise your HDL, the good cholesterol, as you may have learned from advocates of the "Mediterranean diet," which recommends a daily glass of wine for a healthy heart. However, drinking too much alcohol can increase your triglyceride levels and cause liver damage. Alcohol should not be your main defense against CHD.

In addition, the following are risk factors for CHD on their own:

- cigarette smoking
- high blood pressure
- diabetes

What are the benefits of lowering cholesterol?

Several research studies have been conducted to see whether lowering your cholesterol leads to a reduction in the number of heart attacks. In patients who already had CHD, lowering cholesterol clearly prevents second heart attacks and lowers the risk of dying from one. For patients with diabetes in these studies, the benefits of lowering cholesterol are even more dramatic. The same holds true even for people without previous CHD. One major study followed 4,000 patients for 5 years. They found that by lowering LDL with a group of drugs called *statins*, there was a 42% reduction in the number of deaths from heart attacks and a 37% reduction in the chance of having a heart attack.

What does your cholesterol mean to you?

Because diabetes puts you at greater risk for CHD, you want your cholesterol levels to be as close to normal as possible. Your total cholesterol level should be less than 200 mg/dl. Your HDL should be 45 mg/dl or more, the higher the better on this one. **If you have diabetes,** your LDL should be less than 100 mg/dl. Triglycerides should be less than 150 (Table 6-1). The best way to achieve desirable blood fat levels is with a balanced meal plan and daily exercise. If nutrition therapy and exercise do not lower LDL enough, you'll probably need drug therapy as well.

What changes can you make in your diet?

Changes in diet help reduce cholesterol and are one of the most effective means of reducing your weight. The best—and perhaps only—way to get a meal plan that fits you and your lifestyle is to see a registered dietitian (RD) and work together.

You need to reduce the amounts of saturated fat and cholesterol in your diet—and perhaps eat more monounsaturated fat.

Table 6-1. Desirable Cholesterol Levels

Type	Cholesterol Level (mg/dl)
Total cholesterol	<200
HDL (for men)	>45
(for women)	>55
LDL	<100
Triglycerides	<150

> means greater than
< means less than

How does weight control and exercise affect your cholesterol level?

Physical activity helps in reducing weight, increases the good HDL levels, and improves blood glucose and blood pressure levels. Weight loss of 5–10 pounds can lower your cholesterol level another 5–10%. See chapter 20.

When will your physician begin drug treatment?

If your LDL level remains above your goal, despite your best efforts at meal planning and exercise for 6 months, then drug treatment is considered. You must continue with a good diet and exercise program even when you begin drug therapy. These drugs can have side effects, and you should be closely followed by your physician. The drug classes that are commonly used are statins, bile acid resins, nicotinic acid, fibric acid derivatives, and hormones.

Statins

These drugs inhibit the enzyme that controls the rate at which cholesterol is produced by the liver. They also improve the ability of the liver to remove LDL cholesterol from the blood. They apparently stabilize the plaque that lines the arteries, helping to prevent ruptures that lead to clots and heart attacks.

Currently, there are five statin drugs in the U.S. market: lovastatin (Mevacor), pravastatin (Pravachol), simvastatin (Zocor), fluvastatin (Lescol), and atorvastatin (Lipitor). All are equally effective in bringing LDL levels down by about 20–60%. These drugs are given as a single dose at bedtime. Effects are seen in about 4–6 weeks, which is why your blood test should be repeated at about this time. Serious side effects are rare. Mild gastrointestinal symptoms, including abdominal cramps, gas, and constipation, usually go away after the first few weeks. Periodic lab tests are done to watch for changes in liver function. Rarely, some people may develop soreness and weakness of muscles. If this develops, you must stop your medication immediately and see your doctor.

Bile acid resins

These agents bind cholesterol in the intestines, and this combination is then eliminated in the stool. The bile acid resins lower LDL cholesterol by about 10–20%. Cholestyramine and colestipol are the two main drugs available in this class. They can be combined with statins for an additive effect on cholesterol reduction. Their greatest advantage is their safety profile, because they are not absorbed into your system. Bothersome side effects include constipation, bloating, and gas. These side effects can be avoided by taking the drug with meals and with large quantities of water. They can also cause your triglyceride levels to increase, so this will need to be watched. In addition to binding to cholesterol, bile acid resins interfere with the absorption of other medications taken at the same time. The other medications should be taken at least 1 hour before or 4–6 hours after the resin.

Nicotinic acid

Nicotinic acid is often avoided because it increases blood glucose levels. It is a B vitamin and has several beneficial effects, such as causing a 10–20% reduction in LDL cholesterol and a

20–50% reduction in triglyceride levels. It also raises HDL levels by about 15–30%. This drug is inexpensive and available without prescription. Because of potential side effects, don't use it without a doctor's supervision. The immediate-release form is preferred, and start the dose low and raise it slowly. A common side effect is flushing, which can be reduced by taking aspirin first. Discuss this with your doctor.

Fibric acid derivatives

Gemfibrozil (Lopid) is the fibric acid derivative available in the U.S. and is mainly effective in lowering triglyceride levels by about 20–50%.

Hormones

Estrogen replacement raises HDL, lowers LDL, eliminates fat from the bloodstream, increases blood flow throughout the body, and helps keep blood vessels flexible. So it is offered to postmenopausal women who do not have breast cancer or a history of blood clots. Estrogen does have side effects. High doses are associated with increased chance of breast or uterine cancer. If a woman has her uterus, she also needs to take progesterone. Estrogen can cause the blood to clot more easily, putting you at increased risk for a stroke. With low doses, 0.625 mg or less, this is not a problem. The chance for stroke is higher in women with high blood pressure and those who smoke. Hormone therapy works for some women and doesn't work for others. It can cause extremely high triglyceride levels in some people. Women on hormonal therapy should be watched for this, because it can cancel out the other benefits for your heart. Discuss whether hormone therapy would be a good choice for you with your health care provider.

Aruna Venkatesh, MD, and Laurinda M. Poirier, RN, MPH, CDE, contributed to this chapter.

7

Stroke

Case Study

A 65-year-old woman with a history of type 2 diabetes, hypertension, and high cholesterol went to her physician for an episode of "drooping" of the right side of her face, weakness in her right arm, and difficulty with her speech that lasted 15 minutes earlier that day. She reported a blood glucose level of 180 mg/dl after the episode. Her physician told her that he was glad she came for evaluation so quickly. He listened to the carotid arteries in her neck and her heart and performed a neurological examination. He heard a left carotid bruit (a soft, whooshing sound) over the artery in her neck. He recommended further testing, including a carotid artery ultrasound; a complete blood evaluation that included blood glucose, cholesterol, and triglycerides; and a brain computed tomography (CT) scan. He started her on aspirin, which can prevent clotting.

Diabetes increases your risk of having an ischemic stroke. An ischemic stroke is caused by a lack of blood supply to an area of the brain because of blockage of a blood vessel either in or leading to the brain. Your risk of brain hemorrhage is not higher because you have diabetes, so this chapter deals specifically with ischemic stroke. Diabetes does increase your risk of ischemic stroke by approximately two to three times. This increased risk of stroke is present whether you have type 1 or type 2 diabetes and regardless of other risk factors, such as high blood pressure.

People with diabetes tend to have more severe disabilities after stroke, a higher frequency of another stroke, and a higher risk of death after stroke than the general population. However, your risk of stroke can be reduced by knowing the warning signs and by identifying risk factors other than diabetes that you can do something about. There are medications and a surgical procedure called *carotid endarterectomy* that can be used to reduce the risk of stroke in appropriate situations.

What are the signs and symptoms of stroke?

The brain requires a constant blood supply circulated from the heart to the brain arteries. When there is an interruption in the blood supply to an area of the brain, dysfunction of that part of the brain occurs. There are certain warning signs and symptoms that indicate that a temporary (transient ischemic attack, or TIA) or permanent (stroke) lack of blood supply is occurring in the brain.

In approximately 20% of people who go on to have a stroke, there is a preceding TIA that is a clear warning sign of a possible impending stroke, as in the case study. A TIA usually lasts 5–15 minutes and then resolves. It differs from a stroke in one regard, and that is the short, reversible duration of the symptoms. A TIA is an important sign to pay attention to because if a person is treated after it occurs, the risk of a subsequent stroke is reduced.

There are typical warning signs of a TIA or stroke (Table 7-1). One of these signs is sudden weakness or numbness of the face, arm, or leg, usually on one side of the body. Rarely, there may be involvement of both sides of the body at the same time. The weakness may be described as heaviness or clumsiness of the arm and/or leg. There may be weakness

The Uncomplicated Guide to Diabetes Complications

Table 7-1. Warning Signs of a Stroke

- Sudden weakness or numbness of the face, arm, or leg on one side of the body

- Sudden dimness or loss of vision, particularly in one eye

- Loss of speech or trouble talking or understanding speech

- Unexplained dizziness, unsteadiness, or sudden falls, especially with the presence of any of the above symptoms

- Sudden, severe headaches with no apparent cause

of one side of the face, often described by the person as "drooping." There may be sudden dimness or loss of vision, particularly in one eye. This may be described as a "fog," "haze," or "scum" over the eye. Loss of vision may progress from the top to the bottom of the vision in one eye. Individuals may have trouble pronouncing words clearly. Some have trouble understanding words that are spoken, trouble expressing themselves, or difficulty in both areas. There may be difficulty reading or writing. Sudden onset of spinning dizziness (vertigo), unsteadiness of walking, or rarely, a sudden fall can be warning symptoms of an impending stroke. These symptoms may be seen along with visual dimming or loss in both eyes, double vision, or slurred speech. Finally, a sudden, severe headache with no other apparent cause can be a stroke warning symptom. Headaches accompany ischemic stroke approximately 20% of the time.

What are the causes of stroke in a person with diabetes?

Stroke can be divided into ischemic stroke and hemorrhagic stroke. An ischemic stroke is the most common type of stroke, accounting for approximately 80–85% of all strokes. This type occurs when there is blockage of blood flow to the brain due to blockage of an artery or arteries (Figure 7-1). There can be many reasons for an artery being blocked, the most common of which is *atherosclerosis*. Atherosclerosis occurs more commonly, advances more rapidly, and is present at a younger age in people with diabetes.

Another cause of ischemic stroke, called *cardioembolism*, is often due to the development of a clot in one of the chambers of the heart that breaks loose and lodges in an artery of the brain. Other conditions that contribute to this type of

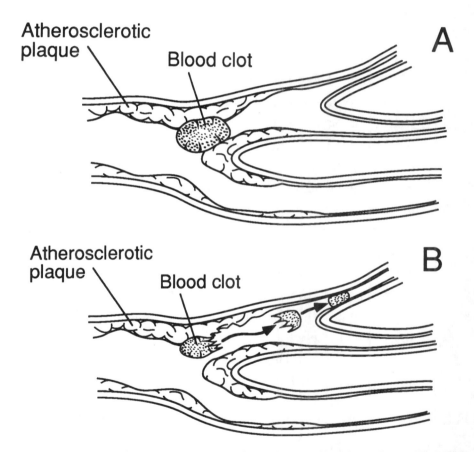

Figure 7-1A. In an area of atherosclerotic narrowing of a blood vessel, a blood clot can form and block off the blood vessel, often leading to a stroke. **B.** A blood clot can originate in the area of an atherosclerotic plaque or it can travel from the heart to the blood vessel. A piece of the clot can break off and lodge in a smaller artery, causing a stroke.

stroke are atrial fibrillation (an irregular rhythm of the heart due to rapid and ineffective beating of the atria of the heart) and history of heart disease, such as a prior heart attack, history of rheumatic fever with heart abnormalities, or congestive heart failure. In a person with diabetes, a heart attack which may go unrecognized by the individual, or a heart that is not contracting properly can lead to this type of stroke.

Another cause of stroke in people with diabetes is having something wrong with the blood. There may be abnormalities in the way the blood clots caused by changes in clotting factors, platelet stickiness and clumping, or the way red blood cells change their shape as they travel through the blood vessels. The end result is that the red blood cells can clot more easily than normal, seen especially in people with diabetic kidney disease (chapter 9).

How does your physician diagnose stroke and determine the cause?

A diagnosis is made on the basis of the sudden onset of symptoms. Testing to detect a stroke includes a brain CT (or CAT) scan or magnetic resonance imaging (MRI) of the brain. A CT scan of the brain quickly creates several images of the brain to help the doctor determine whether the stroke is caused by bleeding (hemorrhage) or blockage (ischemia). MRI produces a three-dimensional image of the brain without the use of radiation. This test can identify small areas of stroke in places the CT may not show, such as the brain stem, cerebellum, and deep in the brain. Newly developed MRI techniques can detect ischemic brain tissue within the first 60 minutes after the stroke begins. An MRI takes longer than a CT to perform. Some people after stroke can't do it either because of their illness or because of claustrophobia in the MRI chamber.

A CT is the usual test that is done immediately after a stroke to determine whether there is bleeding, which would change the way the doctor manages you after stroke. A carotid artery scan is an ultrasound of the neck arteries that can determine whether there is narrowing or total blockage of the carotid arteries in the neck. Cardiac testing may be done, including an electrocardiogram (ECG), to check for an abnormal cardiac rhythm, or an echocardiogram, which is an ultrasound of the heart done to check for any clots in the chambers of the heart or other abnormalities that could be the source of a stroke. In people with diabetes, blood tests for glucose, cholesterol, and triglycerides are particularly important. Low blood glucose (hypoglycemia) can sometimes mimic a stroke or cause a seizure with paralysis. This usually resolves quickly after the low blood glucose is treated, but in some cases, the symptoms may last for several days. Extremely high BG and HHS can be mistaken for a stroke as the person becomes disoriented and confused (chapter 1). The purpose of the basic tests is to try to determine a cause of the stroke, which directs the physician toward the appropriate treatment to prevent another stroke.

What happens after you have a stroke?

After an acute stroke, you are admitted to the hospital, preferably to a stroke unit under the care of a neurologist. Patients who are treated within 3 hours of ischemic stroke should be considered for tissue plasminogen activator (TPA). TPA is a thrombolytic agent (literally, a substance that dissolves a clot) that is used intravenously. The availability of this drug has placed an increased emphasis on the need for emergency management of stroke. TPA is only for people with ischemic stroke (no brain hemorrhage). There are strict guidelines for the use of TPA after stroke.

It may be necessary to see an endocrinologist, internal medicine physician, or family physician for diabetes or high blood pressure treatment. Depending on the type of neurological impairments that are present after stroke, other health care professionals may be consulted, including a dietitian, speech pathologist, physical therapist, occupational therapist, and recreational therapist. After a stroke, you may need intensive rehabilitation under the care of a physician specializing in physical medicine. It is also important to be evaluated for and quickly treated for any depression that may be present.

How can you prevent an initial or recurrent stroke?

Anyone who wants to prevent a stroke needs to consider lowering their risk factors, trying medical therapy, and/or having surgery.

What are the risk factors that you can't change?

Age

Age is the greatest risk factor for stroke. Almost 75% of strokes occur after age 65. In fact, the risk more than doubles with each decade after age 65.

Gender

Stroke is more common in men than in women until the eighth decade of life. While men are at a greater risk for stroke than women at most ages, stroke continues to be a major killer of women. Women are catching up with men because of factors such as smoking, especially smoking while using birth control pills. Women with diabetes are at higher risk than men with diabetes.

Race

African Americans are approximately 60% more likely than Caucasians to have a stroke. It is likely that both genetic and environmental factors play a role. The presence of obesity in African Americans, Latinos, and American Indians causes their risk of developing diabetes to increase significantly, which may be one factor that leads to an increased stroke risk. Part of the high stroke risk in African American women has been related to a higher prevalence of high blood pressure and diabetes in that group.

Family history

Heredity can play a role in the risk of developing stroke. This is particularly true if many people in your family have high blood pressure, diabetes, or high cholesterol.

What are the risk factors that you can change?

Hypertension

High blood pressure is the major risk factor for stroke. Unfortunately, more than half of the people with hypertension do not even know they have it. High blood pressure is defined as a blood pressure measurement greater than 130/80 mmHg on several different readings. People with diabetes have a 40% higher incidence of hypertension. If hypertension is combined with other risk factors, such as obesity, high blood lipids, smoking, or diabetes, the risk of stroke is greatly increased. Successfully treating hypertension has contributed to the decline in the number of strokes and deaths from strokes in recent years.

High blood lipids

High cholesterol accelerates the development of atherosclerosis, which can lead to stroke.

Cardiac disease

There are many different cardiac diseases that can increase the risk of stroke. Some of the more common are heart attack, congestive heart failure, rheumatic heart disease, artificial heart valves, and atrial fibrillation or other heart-rhythm disturbances.

Tobacco

Cigarette smoking increases the risk of stroke dramatically. Men who smoke have a 40% greater chance of having a stroke than do nonsmokers. Women who smoke have a 60% greater chance of having a stroke compared with nonsmokers. If a woman smokes and uses birth control pills, her risk of stroke is increased 22 times. Smoking or exposure to second-hand tobacco smoke increases the chances of developing atherosclerosis.

Alcohol

Heavy or binge drinking is strongly associated with stroke. Alcohol increases blood pressure levels, which increases the risk of stroke.

Drugs

Drugs including cocaine, LSD, amphetamines, diet pills, and ergot derivatives can increase blood pressure and cause stroke. Substances in the drugs can also have toxic effects on the blood vessels that can lead to stroke. Oral contraceptives have been shown to increase your chances of having a blood clot that could lead to a stroke.

Does good blood glucose control help you prevent a stroke?

We don't know yet. The presence of diabetic complications such as coronary artery disease, heart disease, disease of the blood vessels in the legs (peripheral vascular disease), diabetic kidney disease (nephropathy, microalbuminuria), and disease of the blood vessels in the eyes (retinopathy) has been linked in some studies to a greater stroke risk. That's why it's so important for you to stop smoking and to control your blood pressure and your blood glucose to minimize your risk of stroke (Table 7-2).

Table 7-2. How to Reduce Your Risk of Stroke

- Know the warning signs of stroke and obtain emergency treatment if they occur.

- Pay attention to the modifiable risk factors, including high blood pressure, high cholesterol, and heart disease. Avoid tobacco, alcohol, and recreational drugs.

- See your physician regularly. Follow treatments for high blood pressure and heart disease and any treatment given to you by your physician for prevention of stroke.

What are the medical treatments for stroke?

There are three categories of treatments available for prevention of stroke or recurrent stroke. These include medical therapy to prevent clots, such as aspirin, clopidogrel (Plavix), ticlopidine (Ticlid), or extended release dipyridamole plus aspirin (Aggremox); blood "thinners", such as warfarin (Coumadin); or surgical intervention with a procedure called carotid endarterectomy.

Platelet antiaggregants

Platelet antiaggregants work by preventing blood platelets from sticking together and forming clots. The most commonly used drugs in this category are aspirin and ticlopidine (Ticlid). Aspirin has been used for several decades to reduce the risk of stroke. Studies have shown that aspirin reduces the risk of nonfatal stroke by 30%, the risk of nonfatal heart attack by 30%, and the risk of death by 15% compared with groups taking a placebo. Aspirin has the advantages of being inexpensive, generally safe, and well tolerated by most individuals. The most common side effects are gastrointestinal irritation or bleeding. The dosage recommended by physicians in the U.S. varies between 81 and 1,300 mg/day. The appropriate dose for you should be recommended by your physician. Low doses appear as effective as higher doses and have fewer side effects. In 1998, the FDA recommended a dose of 50 to 325 mg/day. Enteric coated aspirin are best tolerated. If you are allergic to aspirin or cannot tolerate it, inform your doctor to get an alternative medication.

While ticlopidine (Ticlid) differs from aspirin in the way it affects the platelets, the end result is prevention of blood clotting. It is more potent than aspirin. In people with diabetes, ticlopidine has been shown to significantly inhibit platelets from sticking together. It has the added benefit of slowing the progression of background retinopathy. Ticlopidine is more expensive than aspirin.

Some of the side effects with ticlopidine are diarrhea, skin rash, and a reduction in the number of infection-fighting white blood cells in the body, which develops in about 1% of patients and is reversible if it is detected early. For this reason, blood tests to detect this potentially fatal side effect are done every 2 weeks for the first 3 months of therapy.

Anticoagulants

Anticoagulants, or blood thinners, such as heparin or warfarin (Coumadin), are another therapy to prevent stroke or recurring strokes. In general, anticoagulants are used in patients who have strokes caused by cardiac clots that break loose and lodge in the brain arteries.

Anticoagulants are also given when patients fail to respond to platelet antiaggregants. Heparin is given intravenously or by injection for a short period immediately after a stroke to prevent the blood from clotting in an area of tight narrowing of a blood vessel.

Warfarin (Coumadin) prevents the blood from clotting by inhibiting the production of some of the clotting factors in the liver. Warfarin helps prevent stroke in people with atrial fibrillation and mechanical heart valves. It may also be used after some types of heart attack to prevent stroke. It is not uncommon for patients to be given both heparin and warfarin for several days after a stroke, followed by the use of warfarin alone once the desired degree of blood thinning is reached. The main potential side effect of these agents is bleeding, either into the brain or at other sites in the body. The degree of thinning of the blood needs to be carefully and frequently monitored with blood testing. Check with your physician about the foods and medications that can affect the warfarin dose. A study reported in 2001 showed that aspirin offers a slight benefit over Wayfarin for prevention of another stroke.

What is the surgical treatment for stroke?

Carotid endarterectomy is a surgical procedure used to clean out the carotid arteries in the neck. In this procedure, the carotid artery is opened, and the layer of plaque (buildup) in the artery is removed. Recent studies have provided some guidelines for performing carotid endarterectomy. In patients with symptoms, either TIA or mild-to-moderate stroke, surgery is highly beneficial if there is 70–99% narrowing of the carotid artery on the same side as the symptoms. Certain patients with symptomatic 50–69% narrowing of the carotid artery also benefit from the procedure. Carotid endarterectomy is not beneficial for symptomatic patients with less than 50% narrowing or in people with complete (100%) blockage of the carotid artery. This surgical procedure is not recommended for patients who are at a high risk for surgical complications, such as those with poor heart or lung function.

Angioplasty with use of a stent is being studied as a treatment for people with narrowing of the cerebral blood vessels.

This chapter was written by Jose Biller, MD, FACP, and Betsy B. Love, MD.

8

Hypertension

Hypertension means high blood pressure. If you have hypertension and diabetes together, you are at higher risk for heart, blood vessel (cardiovascular), and kidney disease.

Mr. LJ is a 43-year-old African-American senior executive who was sent by his company for a health check-up. A few months ago, he was told that he had elevated blood pressure, but because he was feeling fine, it was not treated. He works very hard in a stressful environment. His typical day starts around 8:00 A.M. after a traditional American breakfast of eggs, bacon, and buttered toast. He is so busy that he hardly has time for lunch and usually eats a bag of potato chips or a king-sized candy bar. He finishes work around 7:00 P.M. and spends the evenings with his family having a large dinner and watching TV. He gets little exercise, traveling by car and using the elevator at the office. Mr. LJ smokes a pack of cigarettes daily. He enjoys drinking alcohol but does not use any other recreational drugs. Fortunately, he has not had any major medical illnesses in the past. Both his mother and father have hypertension and diabetes, and his father has had a major heart attack from which he almost died. Mr. LJ is 5 feet 8 inches tall and weighs 250 pounds.

DR. JR: Your blood pressure reading today is high. You told me that a few months ago another doctor recorded high readings. Before I say that you have hypertension, I would like to confirm at least two more readings, a week apart.

MR. LJ: I have heard that some people have high blood pressure only in the doctor's office. Is that what is happening to me?

DR. JR: That is called "white coat hypertension," where people have high blood pressure readings in the doctor's office but normal readings at home. We need to measure your blood pressure at home several times. I will lend you a blood pressure monitor and stethoscope and teach you and your wife how to use them. Then I will see you in a week. With your medical and family history and your lifestyle, you are at risk for high blood pressure, diabetes, elevated blood cholesterol and lipids, and cardiovascular disease, which are all serious diseases. You will have the laboratory screening tests for these. The results should be available the next time we meet.

One week later

DR. JR: Welcome back, Mr. LJ. I have the results of your home blood pressure readings and lab tests. You do indeed have hypertension. Your blood chemistries indicate that you may also have diabetes and high cholesterol.

MR. LJ: Is this a common problem?

DR. JR: Yes. There are approximately 16 million people with diabetes in the U.S. and 30–40 million people with hypertension. Nearly 3 million people have both diseases. You are one of them. So you see, this is a common problem. The causes are both hereditary and environmental. As people age, they are more likely to develop both hypertension and type 2 diabetes. When we consider race, African Americans are almost twice as likely to have diabetes and hypertension, and Mexican Americans are three times more likely to have them than the general population.

MR. LJ: What causes hypertension in people with diabetes?

DR. JR: Hypertension in people with diabetes is usually *essential hypertension* (no cause is found). This is particularly true of type 2 diabetes. We do know that between 35 and 75% of all diabetic complications result from hypertension. It is well worth your time to check what causes yours. Hardening of the arteries, or *atherosclerosis* (the process of cholesterol building up on the blood vessel wall), may narrow the arteries supplying the kidneys. This causes high blood pressure, called *renovascular hypertension*, which is potentially correctable.

MR. LJ: When do you say a person has hypertension?

DR. JR: Hypertension is not diagnosed on a single measurement but on high readings on at least two occasions, a week apart. The American Diabetes Association suggests an average of greater than 80 mmHg diastolic or a systolic blood pressure of greater than 130 mmHg for a diagnosis of hypertension.

MR. LJ: Once you have established that a patient with diabetes has hypertension, what next?

DR. JR: I ask the patient the following questions:
1. Tell me what medications, prescribed and over the counter, you are taking. I want to see whether any of these might contribute to high blood pressure or diabetes. Over-the-counter medications that may raise blood pressure include certain pain medications like ibuprofen, cold and sinus remedies, appetite suppressants, and some drugs used in treating depression.

2. Do you have abnormal blood cholesterol or lipid levels? What were your previous test results?
3. Do you smoke cigarettes?
4. Do you have heart disease, stroke, kidney disease, or eye disease? Have you ever suffered a heart attack? Have you ever had a cardiac (heart) stress test? If so, what were the results?
5. Do other family members have heart disease, hypertension, diabetes, or kidney disease?
6. Do you get cramps in the calves of your legs when you walk short distances?
7. Describe your dietary habits. Do you add salt to prepared foods? Do you consume a lot of canned foods and processed meats? These usually contain large amounts of salt, which raises blood pressure in some salt-sensitive people. Describe your use of alcohol.
8. Do you exercise? If so, what kind? How often?
9. Have you gained or lost weight recently? How much weight and why do you think you lost it?
10. Do you have numbness or tingling in your hands or feet?
11. Have you had any episodes of impotence? Have you had frequent urinary tract infections? Are you unable to empty your bladder when urinating?
12. Do you become dizzy when you stand up?

For already established patients, I ask:
13. How long have you had diabetes and hypertension?
14. What treatments have you received in the past? How did you respond to them? List any side effects you had.
15. Have you been told you have leakage of albumin or protein in the urine?

16. When was your last eye exam? What was the
    result?

MR. LJ: You said you would perform a physical exam.
What are you looking for?

DR. JR: Apart from recording your height and weight, I
would like to measure your blood pressure when you are
standing, sitting, and lying down on your back two or more
separate times (at different visits). This is because there is a
greater variability in blood pressure measurements in people
with diabetes. It will also give me an opportunity to determine whether you are one of those patients whose blood
pressure drops when they stand up. The condition is called
orthostatic hypotension and is especially difficult to treat.
Also, some medications used to treat hypertension may
cause orthostatic hypotension as a side effect, particularly in
people who have diabetes.

I will then examine your neck for distended veins, which
may signify heart failure. I will listen with my stethoscope
on your neck (on both sides of your windpipe) for a bruit—
the sound of blood flowing through narrowed neck arteries
that supply blood to the brain. This gives a clue about the
presence of vascular (blood vessel) disease. Then I will use
a hand-held ophthalmoscope to examine the retinas of your
eyes, and I will check those blood vessels for evidence of
disease resulting from diabetes and/or hypertension.

I will carefully examine your heart for enlargement and
other effects of hypertension, such as hypertrophy (thickening of the wall due to excess work) and failure (inability to
cope with excess demand). I will listen to your lungs to
check for the congestion that accompanies heart failure. I
will listen to your abdomen for bruits (as in the neck). These
sounds come from narrowed renal arteries (arteries that
supply the kidneys). I will check for masses in the flank
areas (to detect enlarged kidneys, which may suggest poly-

cystic [containing many cysts] kidneys) and distended urinary bladder. Diabetes can affect the nerves to the bladder (autonomic nervous system disease). (See chapters 9 and 12.)

I will carefully examine your feet to detect diminished or absent pulses, which suggest peripheral vascular disease (small blood vessel disease; chapter 10), and swelling of the feet and legs (*edema*, caused by fluid building up in the tissues), which may suggest you have heart or kidney failure or side effects from some medications. I will check your nervous system for nerve damage. Peripheral nerve disease with numbness and tingling in the feet is confirmed by loss of feeling. A sensitive method of testing for this is to use a vibrating tuning fork at the base of the big toe. I'll also use a monofilament to test your ability to feel a light touch. We'll do these tests every time I see you.

The results of my examination may show a correctable cause for hypertension. These results can include flank masses, suggesting enlarged polycystic kidney disease; bruits heard especially in the diastolic (the relaxation period of the heart) phase; or bruits heard in the abdomen, suggesting high blood pressure in the blood vessels in the kidneys. I do not find any organ damage. Therefore, I assume that you have not had high blood pressure for long

MR. LJ: Could you explain what tests you performed?

DR. JR: Before I begin a treatment and at the time of diagnosis, I request a series of blood tests that include serum creatinine (a marker of kidney function), TSH (a thyroid test), electrolyte levels that may point to hypertension caused by excess production of certain hormones, a CBC (complete blood count) to check for anemia, and a glycated hemoglobin (A1C) to measure your blood sugar levels over the past 2–3 months. A fasting blood lipids profile to detect abnormalities in your cholesterol levels (cholesterol, HDL,

LDL, and triglycerides) is also important for patients with diabetes and hypertension.

A complete urinalysis will detect any proteinuria (protein leaking into the urine) or other problems. This will include a 24-hour collection of urine to check for small amounts of protein (called *albumin*) that might not show up in the single urine sample.

We will repeat some of these tests 6–12 weeks after treatment is begun to see the effects of medication, especially on blood lipids. These are tests that you should have at least yearly, but the type of tests and how often you have them should be based on the damage to your organs and how you respond to the selected treatments. You may need other specialized tests or consultations.

MR. LJ: Will I need to see any specialists?

DR. JR: Having determined that you do not have organ damage, I'll refer you to an ophthalmologist for now. I recommend this for adult patients when they are diagnosed with diabetes (see chapter 4).

I am also going to have you see a registered dietitian (RD). You will need a carefully planned diet because you have diabetes, hypertension, and elevated blood lipids (loosely termed *cholesterol*). The RD will help you develop a meal plan with foods you choose for meals and snacks that will supply the total calories you need and help you lose weight.

I also want you to see Ms. DF, a registered nurse clinician specially educated and certified in diabetes education (a certified diabetes educator, or CDE). She will teach you how to check your blood glucose and blood pressure at home and help you deal with specific situations. You can call her when you have questions.

MR. LJ: What symptoms do patients with hypertension usually have? Why didn't I have any symptoms?

DR. JR: Most patients with hypertension have no symptoms. You are a classic example. By the time symptoms appear, organ damage has often set in. The symptoms are from the damaged organs themselves. Physicians have to be on the lookout and screen for hypertension periodically. This is usually done during annual physical exams, employment physicals, or ordinary visits to health providers for some other cause such as an acute illness. Certainly, if a patient has a family history of heart disease, kidney disease, diabetes, or hypertension, routine screening is necessary.

MR. LJ: How do I go about managing my problems?

DR. JR: There are several phases to managing your health problems. You'll need to make some lifestyle changes. As I told you earlier, you have diabetes, hypertension, and elevated blood lipids. What you eat is a key factor in your management. You are overweight, and losing weight plays a major role in controlling all three problems. You'll be encouraged to know that you will start seeing significant benefits even after losing only a few pounds. You do not have to reach an ideal body weight to see results.

Exercise is as important as food. The type of exercise should be aerobic—walking, jogging, bicycling, swimming, or rowing. You should not do high-intensity exercises, such as weight lifting done with a bearing-down motion or holding your breath, which increase the strain on the heart and elevate blood pressure. (You probably can lift light weights and build strength with more repetitions, but get instruction from a qualified teacher.) You don't want more harm than good to come from your exercise. It is important to get medical advice before you begin an exercise program. I'd like you to see Dr. MM, a cardiologist and exercise physiologist, who may perform an exercise stress test to check how your heart performs during exercise. Remember, you should start slowly, progress gradually, and report any symptoms such as chest pain and shortness of breath immediately. Don't just rely on the exercise test results.

MR. LJ: What do you mean by lifestyle changes?

DR. JR: Diet and exercise are the most important ways that we define our lifestyle—the way we choose to live. Changing these two significantly affects your health. Other powerful lifestyle changes are stopping cigarette smoking completely, using alcohol in moderation, and reducing stress. If you make all of these changes, you'll take control of all three medical conditions and prevent complications.

MR. LJ: I have read somewhere about nonpharmacological treatments. What are those?

DR. JR: The name means treatment without the use of drugs. This is actually a different way to describe those lifestyle changes, such as avoiding tobacco and eating less fat. I usually try nonpharmacological treatment alone for a period of 3 months if the initial blood pressure readings are not very high (generally lower than 160/95 mmHg).

However, if you have organ damage, risk factors like elevated blood lipids, diabetes, cigarette smoking, obesity, sedentary lifestyle, or family history of premature cardiovascular disease, I may prescribe drug therapy at the time of diagnosis. You fall into this category. However, I strongly recommend that you make the lifestyle changes, too. If you succeed with nonpharmacological measures, you'll require smaller amounts of medication to control your blood pressure. You may also reduce side effects from the drugs and find it's easier to take them. Lifestyle changes will help increase your chances for successful step-down therapy (reducing dosage and/or number of drugs) after your blood pressure has been well controlled for more than 1 year on at least four consecutive office visits.

MR. LJ: Since you have made it clear that I will need drug therapy, I'm curious about how you choose the right drug combination for me. Are specific drugs indicated for specific patient groups? Please explain.

DR. JR: The Joint National Committee for Hypertension has extensively reviewed several treatment approaches to hypertension. The combination of hypertension and diabetes carries a greater risk of target organ damage than does either disease alone. That's why there are special qualifications for when to use hypertension drug therapy for people with diabetes.

1. Patients with diabetes and hypertension who have blood pressure of 140/90 mmHg or higher are candidates for drug therapy to reduce blood pressure to 130/80 mmHg or less.
2. The presence of complicating kidney disease limits drug choices because of the effects of each drug on kidney function and diabetic nephropathy.
3. Some drugs can upset blood glucose and blood lipid levels.
4. Orthostatic hypotension is common in people with diabetes and needs to be remembered when choosing which drugs to use.

In clinical trials, only beta blockers and diuretics have been shown to decrease death from cardiovascular disease. I tend to use beta blockers only under special circumstances, for example, in patients with diabetes and hypertension who have angina or after a heart attack, where it can prevent sudden death. Diuretics are better known as water pills. There are several classes of these drugs depending on how and where in the kidneys they act. I won't go into the complex actions of these drugs. Generally, there is no reason to use diuretics except thiazides for the treatment of hypertension. Thiazide diuretics in low doses (25 mg/day or less) have acceptable side effects and generally work for people with diabetes. Because diuretics can cause potassium loss, you would need frequent tests of blood potassium and may need a potassium supplement.

Another recommended class of drugs for patients with diabetes and hypertension is the *converting enzyme inhibitors*. These agents are based on the principle that there is an enzyme chiefly in the lung (but also in other tissues) called angiotensin-converting enzyme, or simply ACE. ACE converts angiotensin I to angiotensin II, which has strong effects on blood vessels, constricting them and elevating blood pressure. By successfully blocking (inhibiting) the action of this enzyme, these drugs reduce blood pressure. That's why they are called ACE inhibitors. They also have several other beneficial effects. Most important, they reduce proteinuria and slow the progression of diabetic kidney disease. They do not affect blood glucose control and do not raise blood lipids, but these drugs are not without side effects. ACE inhibitors in rare instances can worsen kidney function in patients with narrowing of both renal arteries. Therefore, we would need to monitor serum creatinine and potassium. We must take care when combining therapy with diuretics because the drop in blood pressure can be deep. Cough is a common side effect of ACE inhibitors.

Another class of drugs to treat hypertension is the calcium-channel blockers, also known as calcium antagonists. **Generally, they should not be used for people with diabetes.**

A class of drugs called alpha blockers has also been recommended. Like beta receptors, there are alpha receptors in the blood vessels. Blocking alpha receptors makes the blood vessels relax, thereby decreasing their resistance and lowering blood pressure. These drugs do not affect blood glucose levels. They may also have a beneficial effect on blood lipids. Caution is needed when beginning these agents, because the very first dose can cause a sharp drop in blood pressure. I usually warn patients of this and start them on the lowest dose. I ask the patient to take the medication at bedtime and advise caution when rising. These drugs may also help patients with enlargement of the prostate and difficult urination by relaxing the urethra. This is an example of the two-for-one concept—a drug is selected not only for its effect on blood pressure but also for its effect on coexisting diseases or symptoms.

A newer class of agents, the *angiotensin II receptor blockers,* block the effect of angiotensin II and are very effective in lowering blood pressure. They significantly reduce proteinuria, improve blood lipid levels, and don't cause side effects like coughs. There is no dosage adjustment necessary for patients with kidney disease, and needing to take them only once a day improves the likelihood of people remembering to take them.

MR. LJ: All this talk about drugs makes me wonder how much lifestyle changes can reduce blood pressure.

DR. JR: In a study called TOMHS (Trial of Mild Hypertension Study), lifestyle changes alone reduced average blood pressure from 141/91 to 130/83 mmHg for 234 participants after 1 year.

MR. LJ: Would you recommend lifestyle changes for normal people?

DR. JR: Yes. It would make everyone healthier and happier. I would recommend lifestyle changes to everyone, especially those with blood pressure in the high-normal range (systolic 130–139 and diastolic 80–89 mmHg) to keep them from developing high blood pressure in the future.

MR. LJ: You mentioned earlier that the presence of diabetes and hypertension worsens the target organ damage more than either disease does alone. Could you explain this with specific examples of the target organs?

DR. JR: I'm glad you asked. Let's take cardiovascular disease. The risk to your heart and blood vessels is doubled when you have diabetes and hypertension. This includes coronary heart disease (which produces heart attacks), heart failure, and peripheral vascular disease, causing poor circulation in arms and legs, which can end in amputation. The risk of strokes is increased by two to four times in people with diabetes. Hypertension increases the risk by six times. Thus, the risk of stroke is substantial when you have both diseases.

Eyes are another target. Eye disease (retinopathy) can be affected by diabetes and hypertension. Patients with both diseases are definitely at higher risk for optic nerve damage and glaucoma. Systolic blood pressure (the top number) is a predictor of the frequency of it happening, and diastolic blood pressure (the bottom number) predicts the progression of retinopathy. Retinopathy is twice as likely to occur when the average systolic blood pressure is 145 versus 125 mmHg. Diabetic retinopathy is the most frequent cause of new cases of blindness in American adults aged 20–74 years. Good control of hypertension can go a long way in preserving eyesight.

Remember how the kidneys can be damaged, a disease called diabetic nephropathy. Hypertension speeds up the progression of this complication. Remember that control of hypertension along with good blood glucose control can prevent the progression of nephropathy. So, you see that controlling hypertension is a key factor in preventing some of the dreaded complications of diabetes.

MR. LJ: Some of my friends who take medicines for blood pressure have problems with their sex life. I am skeptical of taking medications because I feel it may destroy my harmonious family life.

DR. JR: I know you're concerned about the side effects of the drugs, but the diseases themselves can cause sexual problems in both men and women. Certainly, hypertension, neuropathy, poor circulation, and psychological problems can cause impotence, impaired ejaculation, or decreased libido in men (chapter 17). In women, these complications can result in decreased vaginal lubrication, decreased libido, and difficulty in achieving an orgasm (chapter 18). Lowering your blood pressure can help prevent all these complications.

Certainly, your concern is valid. The drugs can have this side effect, but it should not stop you from taking them for now. Keep an open mind and if this problem does occur in the future, we can adjust your medication to minimize the problem.

MR. LJ: That is very reassuring. Now that I am ready to take on treatment for my conditions, what should I do to be sure that my treatments are successful? Why do treatment programs fail and what can be done to make them successful?

DR. JR: Maintaining a long-term effective treatment regimen is not possible without continued commitment by you, your family, and me. Aside from your primary physician— me—other health care practitioners, such as nurses, pharmacists, podiatrists, dietitians, and ophthalmologists, can play vital roles in education and support of you and your family.

I would encourage you to master the skills you need for self-care and follow the treatment plan we are going to develop together. I'll try to make the instructions simple and clear. I'll also write them down so that you can refer to them later.

MR. LJ: Why does a program fail?

DR. JR: The major reason is that patients don't make lifestyle changes or take their drugs. Sometimes this is because of the cost of the drug, unclear instructions, instructions not being written down, not enough patient education, or the physician trying to dictate to the patients instead of treating them as partners in decision making.

One helpful strategy is to have the patient sign a written contract with realistic short-term goals. The doctor and patient can review them periodically, taking care not to be judgmental if the program isn't working. Patience and perseverance are the rules for success.

By the same token, a successful patient-education program should be tailored to the patient and be culturally sensitive. The diabetes educator must pay attention to the ethnic, religious, and regional issues of the patients. Adults need hands-on, active learning. And the family should be involved at every stage. They can help record the results of blood glucose and blood pressure monitoring in a simple-to-use log book. The log book should be reviewed periodically with the provider to make treatment decisions. Providers should keep patients aware of available community resources and programs at workplaces and health care institutions.

MR. LJ: Speaking of home monitoring. What kind of blood pressure instrument do you recommend for use at home? How do I interpret the numbers?

DR. JR: The "gold standard" for blood pressure measurement is the mercury sphygmomanometer, but it is more difficult to learn to use. There are new electronic models with increasing degrees of sophistication. You want a monitor that is consistent, accurate, easy to use, and affordable. Your machine should be checked against the one in my office periodically to make sure your home monitoring results are accurate. Whatever instrument you choose to use, make sure you choose an appropriate cuff size, place the arm at the level of the heart, and are well rested before taking measurements. Remember that blood pressure readings vary at different times of the day. In addition, physical activity, stress, caffeine, tobacco, and alcohol can influence readings. Be honest when you write down the results, because you cannot fool the target organs! It is better to stay away from electronic finger models because there are more factors that can interfere and give false readings.

MR. LJ: Are there any separate guidelines for managing patients with diabetes and hypertension among special groups?

DR. JR: I would consider children, pregnant women, and elderly people as special groups. I'll tell you about the elderly patient with diabetes and hypertension. The other two groups are dealt with by specialists. I had mentioned earlier that both diabetes and hypertension increase with age. The elderly patient benefits as much as, if not more than, his younger counterpart from treatment of hypertension. This is true even of the very old (over 85 years) and for elevation of either diastolic or systolic blood pressure.

Elderly patients sometimes have difficulty in metabolizing drugs (because of alterations in blood flow to the liver and decreased kidney function), can't afford drugs, or fail to take their drugs because of decreased memory and dementia. It is wise to start with the lowest drug dose and cautiously and slowly increase it. Drugs have longer duration of action in the elderly than in other groups. Orthostatic hypotension can be a problem, but wearing elastic stockings may help.

MR. LJ: I've heard that some patients have elevated systolic blood pressure alone. Do you recommend treating them?

DR. JR: When such patients (systolic blood pressure higher than 160 mmHg but diastolic blood pressure lower than 90 mmHg) are treated, they can benefit in cardiovascular health. I recommend a small dose of a thiazide diuretic at first. These patients are usually elderly and need to be seen frequently. When beginning treatment, they should be watched for orthostatic hypotension, or low blood pressure, on standing up. If a second drug is needed, I recommend an ACE inhibitor. If the elderly patient also has heart failure, the ACE inhibitor will treat both conditions.

MR. LJ: Could you help me better understand the mechanisms underlying these two diseases?

DR. JR: The likelihood of developing both type 2 diabetes and hypertension increases with age, especially in the African-American population. There is a change in body composition that occurs with aging—a significant loss of muscle and an increase in total body fat. The skeletal muscle is mostly responsible for metabolizing carbohydrates, which may explain why diabetes is strikingly high in the elderly. A particular kind of obesity called *abdominal obesity* (as opposed to obesity where the fat is in the hips) is tightly linked to a number of diseases such as diabetes, hypertension, and coronary artery disease. If your waist and hips are about the same size, you're in this group.

Certain minority groups have specific risk factors. African Americans are more sensitive to salt. Genetic factors count, but social and economic factors play significant roles. Factors include diet, exercise, obesity, and insulin resistance. People in lower socioeconomic classes, particularly women, are much more likely to develop obesity, diabetes, and high blood pressure.

MR. LJ: What promise does the future hold for a patient with hypertension and diabetes?

DR. JR: There are some new drugs that lower blood pressure and improve diabetes control called thiazolidinediones or 'glitazones. These drugs increase insulin sensitivity without stimulating the body to produce more insulin. Indeed, these compounds given over a 12-week period decreased insulin resistance, improved blood glucose levels, and lowered blood pressure in obese people who did not have diabetes.

This chapter was written by Venkatraman Rajkumar, MD, and James R. Sowers, MD.

9

Nephropathy

Case study

A 37-year-old woman who has had type 1 diabetes since age 7 noticed ankle swelling and increasing girth over a 6-month period. Over the years, her blood sugar control had only been fair, ranging from 140 to 300 mg/dl. She had high blood pressure (150/95 to 180/105 mmHg). Albuminuria (increasing amounts of albumin, a protein, in her urine) had been showing up in her lab tests for the last 2 years. She recently needed laser therapy for proliferative diabetic retinopathy. Her current lab tests showed large amounts of albumin in her urine. Her serum creatinine was 2.1 mg/dl (normal is less than 1.2 mg/dl). When the kidneys start to fail, the blood creatinine begins to rise. Her physician diagnosed nephrotic syndrome, a condition of protein loss, water retention, and high cholesterol. He prescribed an ACE inhibitor, a medicine that lowers blood pressure and helps preserve kidney function, and a diuretic. A statin drug was included to reduce LDL cholesterol to less than 100. He sent her to an RD for help in following a reduced-fat, limited protein, low-salt diet.

Case study

After 11 years of type 2 diabetes, a 54-year-old, African-American man with high blood pressure (180/110) complained of being unable to concentrate and of constantly feeling cold. Weakness, nausea, a 12-pound weight loss, and itchy skin were also complaints. On physical examination, the patient was found to have advanced renal disease with a serum creatinine of 11.6 mg/dl (normal is less than 1.5 mg/dl. Normal is higher for men than for women). He recently needed laser surgery for diabetic retinopathy, and this supported the diagnosis of advanced diabetic nephropathy. The patient, his wife, and his clergyman met to consider whether dialysis or a kidney transplant was the best option for him. Three brothers and two sisters all offered to donate a kidney.

Today, diabetes is the leading cause of kidney (renal) failure worldwide. The good news is that the more successful you are at managing your diabetes, the longer and healthier your life should be. The bad news is that a longer life span gives some people with diabetes time to develop the "late" complications of diabetes, including kidney failure. That may be why diabetes now accounts for 46% of all new cases of kidney failure. African Americans, Latinos, and American Indians (especially the Pima tribe) are three to five times more likely to have both diabetes and kidney complications. Of people with type 1 diabetes, 30–50% are likely to develop diabetic nephropathy after having diabetes for 40 years. In people with type 2 diabetes, diabetic nephropathy is a bit of a mystery. Damage to their kidneys has become a sign that they are at risk for a stroke or heart attack.

However, ongoing research and improvements in diabetes management have improved the quality of life of all people afflicted with serious kidney disease. In fact, over the past decade, there has been steady improvement in the survival of diabetic kidney failure patients treated by dialysis or a kidney transplant.

What do your kidneys do?

The two kidneys are located in the back of the abdomen on either side of the spine. Each is about the size of an Idaho potato weighing about 1/2 pound, and together they process about one-quarter of the blood pumped by the heart. One kidney can do the work for two, which is why people born with only one kidney or who lose a kidney by trauma, disease, or as a transplant donor have a normal life expectancy. Blood flow through the kidney amounts to about one quart every minute. The kidneys' job is to remove nitrogen-rich end products of protein digestion and water and to maintain a balance of sodium and potassium. The kidneys also manufacture hormones that stimulate the bone marrow to make red blood cells and regulate calcium absorption from the intestines. Like other vital organ systems, renal function has a large reserve capacity.

Each kidney is made up of between 600,000 and nearly 1.5 million subunits called *nephrons*. Specialists in internal medicine who work primarily with diseases of the kidney are called *nephrologists*. Individual nephrons begin with a complex of tiny blood vessel loops called a *glomerulus*, through which blood from the heart is filtered. The blood is delivered by an *arteriole*—a small artery. Blood, minus what was filtered, leaves through another arteriole to return through veins to the heart. The filtrate enters a long path in the nephron called a *tubule*, where it is changed into urine and discharged into the bladder via the *ureters*—tubes connecting the kidneys to the bladder (Figure 9-1).

Disease of the kidney (renal disease) is called *nephropathy*, and people with diabetes have *diabetic nephropathy*. However, not all kidney disease in those who have diabetes is related to diabetes. For example, you may inherit a kidney disorder, have a tumor or enlargement of the prostate gland that obstructs urine flow and puts backup pressure on the kidney,

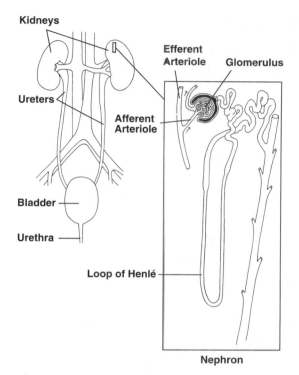

Figure 9-1. The kidneys and urinary system.

or have an infectious disease that affects your kidneys. Certain drugs can also injure kidney function. That is why it is sometimes difficult to determine whether kidney disease is diabetes related or caused by something else.

Who is at risk for developing diabetic nephropathy?

The longer you have diabetes, the more at risk you are for developing diabetic neuropathy. But after 40 years of diabetes, only 30–50% of people with type 1 diabetes develop kidney disease. People whose blood glucose control is not good are more at risk for developing the disease. Some people have a genetic tendency to develop the disease, especially if a near relative has it. People with high blood pressure are more likely to develop nephropathy—and nephropathy makes high blood pressure even worse. Other risk factors include high cholesterol levels, urinary tract infections (UTIs), and smoking.

What are the symptoms of kidney disease?

Unfortunately, kidney disease doesn't have any symptoms until it is pretty far along. That is why laboratory tests need to be done at regular intervals to tell you and your physician how your kidneys are doing before serious symptoms show up.

What are the stages of diabetic kidney disease?

Although not seen in every individual, the stages of diabetic kidney disease have been divided into hyperfiltration, microalbuminuria, nephrotic syndrome, renal insufficiency, and end-stage renal disease.

What is hyperfiltration?

The first stage of diabetic kidney disease has no symptoms and is called *hyperfiltration*. Early in the course of diabetes, in as many as 70% of those with type 1 diabetes and about 33% of those with type 2 diabetes, an above-normal amount of blood passes through the filtering glomeruli in their kidneys. The cause has been linked to long-term high blood glucose levels. Kidney size increases early in the development of diabetic kidney disease. Lowering blood glucose levels can, however, reduce kidney size to normal. A kidney function test called *clearance* may show that you are experiencing hyperfiltration, but that does not mean that your kidneys will get worse. Less than 50% of people who have diabetes and hyperfiltration go on to the later stages of nephropathy.

What is microalbuminuria?

Microalbuminuria is the condition of small amounts of a protein called albumin showing up in your urine. Healthy people have less than 25 mg of albumin in their urine each day. Microalbuminuria (30–300 mg/day) occurs in 4–15% of adults with diabetes, typically in those who have had the disease for at least 5 years. Hyperfiltration may not be present with microalbuminuria. It is important to detect microalbuminuria early because people with type 1 diabetes who have microalbuminuria are more likely to progress to the later stages of kidney disease. People with type 2 diabetes who have it are more likely to have a heart attack or stroke. If you have microalbuminuria, you may prevent or slow the development of more serious conditions for many years by bringing your blood pressure down to normal and by achieving good blood glucose control. A specific laboratory test must be done to find microalbuminuria, because the usual urine dipsticks or clinic tests for protein are not sensitive enough. The first morning specimen of urine is the most reliable. If this test is positive, a 24-hour urine specimen should be checked for total albumin content. The result can be compared with the same test taken after treatment is begun, to see whether there has been improvement. Repeat tests need to be taken because the level of albumin in urine naturally varies from day to day for different reasons. It may also be influenced by exercise.

Although microalbuminuria has no signs or symptoms, we know that there are changes in the small blood vessels of the kidneys that are unique to diabetes and that blood pressure increases in the filters in the kidneys. Microalbuminuria signals the need for treatment with ACE inhibitors or a class of drugs called A2 receptor blockers. ACE inhibitors lower the blood pressure within the glomerulus so that less protein, or albumin, is leaking from the blood into the urine, and they slow the deterioration of kidney function. Indeed, many doctors advise an ACE inhibitor or A2 receptor blocker for every diabetic individual. About 10% of those treated may develop a dry cough or other side effect and have to stop taking it.

What is nephrotic syndrome?

If the injury to the blood filters in the kidneys gets worse, albumin loss in the urine rises to 3,500 mg/day or more and can be measured by a dipstick test. This stage is called dipstick-positive *proteinuria*, or clinical nephropathy. The changes that take place in the kidneys are called the *nephrotic syndrome*.

Because you're losing so much albumin in your urine, the level of albumin in the blood decreases to less than the normal range of about 3.9–4.6 mg/dl. This diminishes the ability of the blood to hold plasma water inside the arteries and capillaries. Water then accumulates in the tissues as *edema* and in the chest (*pleural effusion*), around the heart (*pericardial effusion*), and in the abdomen (*ascites*). These are the areas where you may notice symptoms if the disease has progressed this far. The liver increases albumin synthesis to compensate for the low plasma level. The liver also produces more cholesterol and fats (*hyperlipidemia*), which can cause other health problems. In the nephrotic syndrome, fluid is retained in the body, and water weight may reach 50 pounds. Carrying this much extra water causes fatigue and shortness of breath due to fluid in the chest. People with nephrotic syndrome often note that their shoes don't fit and dresses and pants will not button because of the water weight, and even routine activities are difficult and tiring to complete.

What is renal insufficiency?

This stage is called advanced clinical nephropathy or kidney failure. At this stage, the damaged kidney is no longer able to filter all of the toxins produced daily from the blood or prevent protein from leaking into the urine. Among the protein wastes proposed as toxins are urea, creatinine, uric acid, phenols, and guanidines. Physicians monitor the condition of the kidneys by blood tests measuring either the nitrogen in urea (blood urea nitrogen, or BUN) or the serum creatinine. More precise estimates of remaining kidney function can be obtained by a clearance test of urine and blood together to measure either creatinine or a radioisotope (radioactive chemical) excreted by the kidney. This test often requires a timed urine collection.

Patients have few symptoms until renal function declines to less than 30% and the serum creatinine and BUN levels are higher than normal. When serum creatinine rises above 2.0, the patient should see a nephrologist. Listlessness, loss of appetite, feeling cold, being unable to concentrate, nausea, and itching are common complaints as kidney failure becomes more severe. Anemia is common. Once renal function declines to less than about 15%, symptoms of kidney failure such as skin bruising, intermittent vomiting, weight loss, somnolence during the day and insomnia at night, restless legs, and lethargy may convert a formerly active individual to a chronic invalid. At this stage, less insulin is needed because less insulin is eliminated by the kidneys.

What is end-stage renal disease (ESRD)?

After months to years of renal insufficiency, renal function decreases to the point where life is no longer possible without major therapeutic intervention. Untreated ESRD may induce major swelling of the bowel and fluid collection into the sac surrounding the heart, thereby limiting its ability to pump blood. Muscle cramps and even death may occur when blood potassium rises because potassium cannot be excreted in the urine. High blood potassium levels affect heart function. Patients may also have convulsions. *Uremia*—Greek for "urine in the blood"—is the term applied to ESRD in its last stages. All of the signs and symptoms of uremia can be reversed by dialysis or "cured" by a kidney transplant.

What happens when your kidneys don't work as they should?

When there is injury or disease and kidney function in both kidneys falls to below about 25% of normal for age, sex, and body size, you develop uremia. When this happens, nitrogen-containing compounds build up in your blood and tissues. Then edema—excess fluid in tissues—can be seen and felt in your legs, beneath the skin, and around your eyes, because you are not excreting as much water as you should in your urine. This causes your blood pressure to go up. Hypertension (high blood pressure) is very common in people with diabetes and in people who have uremia. (See chapter 8.)

What can you do to slow or prevent diabetic nephropathy?

The way you can prevent or slow kidney damage is to control high blood pressure; eat a balanced diet that is lower in fats, cholesterol, and protein; and maintain near-normal blood glucose levels.

How does controlling hypertension help?

Early detection and treatment of hypertension (high blood pressure) slows the damage to the kidneys remarkably. The single greatest technique in controlling diabetic kidney complications is to decrease high blood pressure. Hypertension (defined as blood pressure higher than 140/85 mmHg) contributes to continuing loss of kidney function. It is widely felt that people with diabetes who have microalbuminuria or proteinuria should be treated with certain blood pressure–lowering medications, particularly with an ACE inhibitor or A2 receptor blocker, even when they do not have hypertension. Regular testing of blood pressure protects against silent yet dangerous hypertension. At every stage of diabetic kidney disease, having normal blood pressure not only is advisable, but is the mainstay of successful therapy.

How does diet help?

Restricting dietary protein improves the condition of uremic patients and may slow the progression of renal insufficiency. Current practice limits protein intake to 40–60 grams of protein a day. Lowering protein intake from typically excessive amounts to recommended amounts may be helpful in all stages of diabetic nephropathy.

It is equally important to have a diet low in saturated fats and cholesterol. You may need to adjust your diet to unsaturated fats and to take blood cholesterol–lowering medication. This is appropriate at every stage of diabetic nephropathy. A dietitian can offer skilled advice in dealing with your dietary requirements.

How does good blood glucose control help?

Keeping blood glucose levels normal helps prevent or slow the progression of kidney complications for people with type 1 and type 2 diabetes.

What else can harm your kidneys?

Your kidneys may be injured by drugs that you can buy over the counter, such as ibuprofen (Advil, Motrin, and others) and naproxen (Aleve), antibiotics such as cisplatin, and psychiatric medications such as lithium. There are also more than 20 other prescription nonsteroidal anti-inflammatory drugs that will damage your kidneys. If you already have reduced kidney function, the risk of damage from these drugs is greater. If you don't know whether a drug you're going to take will harm your kidneys, ask your physician and pharmacist. You and your physician must weigh the potential harm against the potential benefit of any of these drugs. Fortunately, there are safer substitutes for most of these drugs.

When the dye used for X-ray studies such as angiograms or intravenous pyelograms (IVPs, which evaluate the structure of the kidneys) is injected into your vein or artery, it carries a risk of kidney failure in a few days. This condition is usually reversible but sometimes requires dialysis. If dyes must be used—for example, before urgent coronary artery bypass surgery—you can be given fluids intravenously before and after the procedure and certain drugs, theophylline plus allopurinol, to decrease the likelihood of acute renal failure. Treatment with acetylcystein (Mucomyst) before exposure to radioactive dyes has also been shown to prevent kidney damage.

Finally, one thing inside your body can harm your kidneys. A neurogenic bladder—one that cannot empty urine normally—can make urine back up to the kidneys and cause damage. Infection is common in people with a neurogenic bladder. (See chapter 12.)

What should you do if ESRD happens to you?

Until its later stages, renal disease in diabetes is silent. Other conditions that get worse as kidney function declines divert your attention from ESRD. You may become sleepless, apprehensive, and depressed when you realize that you are faced with what seems to be an unending maze of doctors, procedures, and problems with other major organs. Medical expenses may strain family budgets. At this point, a medical team captain serving as patient advocate, physician coordinator, and friendly advisor can make the difference for you.

What is the treatment for ESRD?

ESRD is treated by repeated dialysis or by a kidney transplant.

What is dialysis?

Dialysis is a process that uses a machine (an artificial kidney) to remove the waste products that have accumulated in the blood. There must be a connection to a blood vessel (vascular access), usually in your forearm, permitting blood to flow to and from the artificial kidney. Typically, *hemodialysis* is performed three times a week for 4–6 hours each time.

Another form of dialysis, called *peritoneal dialysis*, removes wastes from the blood in small blood vessels in the membrane lining your abdominal cavity. After the physician creates a "permanent" access to this area, dialysate can be put into and drained from the abdomen at regular intervals. Continuous ambulatory peritoneal dialysis (CAPD) is the most common of this type of dialysis. During CAPD, approximately 2 liters of dialysate are infused and drained every 4–6 hours by the patient. You do not have to go to the hospital or clinic for this.

For the large majority of people with diabetes—more than 80%—who develop ESRD in the U.S., hemodialysis is the therapy. Approximately 12% of the others will be treated with peritoneal dialysis, and the remaining 8% will receive a kidney transplant. People who are motivated and well-trained are quite successful with peritoneal dialysis. The advantages of CAPD are freedom from a machine, rapid training, minimal cardiovascular stress, and avoidance of the need (as with hemodialysis) for an anti-clotting drug called heparin. Although some physicians call CAPD a first choice treatment for ESRD patients with diabetes, you and your physician should weigh the pros and cons of each before deciding what is best for you (Table 9-1). The disadvantages of CAPD are the need to pay constant attention to fluid exchange, being at constant risk of peritonitis (infection of the lining of the abdomen) that requires hospitalization, and running out of abdominal area to use.

The results of daily hemodialysis are being studied. Reports indicate that patients' blood pressure is lower, there is less anemia, and they have a greater sense of well-being.

Dialysis is not likely to give you the same long-term results as a kidney transplant. Current statistics show that about half of the people with diabetes who start on hemodialysis die within 4 years. This is often from a heart attack because many of these patients also have hypertension and cardiovascular problems. But success rates are improving each year.

Table 9-1. Choices for Uremic Patients with Diabetes

Variable	Peritoneal Dialysis	Hemodialysis	Kidney Transplant
Other serious disease	No limitation	No limitation except for hypotension	Not for patients with cardiovascular disease
Geriatric patients	No limitation	No limitation	Determined by program
Complete rehabilitation	Unlikely, persistent problems	Unlikely, persistent problems	Common as long as transplant functions
Death rate	Higher than for nondiabetic patients	Higher than for nondiabetic patients	About the same as nondiabetic patients
First-year survival	About 80%	About 80%	>90%
Survival to second decade	Undetermined because therapy relatively new	Increasing but rare	About 1 in 5
Progression of complications	Continuing attention to other conditions essential	Persistent problems	Probably reduced in type 1 diabetes by functioning pancreas + kidney. Fewer complications than in dialysis patients.
Special advantage	Can be self-performed. Avoids swings in solute and intravascular volume level.	Can be self-performed. Efficient extraction of solute and water in hours.	Cures uremia. Freedom to travel.
Disadvantage	Peritonitis. Long hours of treatment. More days hospitalized than either hemodialysis or transplant.	Access point is a hazard for clotting, hemorrhage, and infection. Cyclical low blood pressure, weakness.	Cosmetic disfigurement due to drugs given to sustain transplant. Expense for medications can be stress.
Patient acceptance	Variable, usual compliance with passive tolerance for regimen. Burnout after months to years.	Variable, often do not follow dietary, diabetic, or blood pressure guidance.	Enthusiastic during periods of good renal allograft function. Exalted when pancreas proffers euglycemia. Medication noncompliance.
Bias in comparison	Delivered as first choice by enthusiasts, although emerging evidence indicates substantially higher mortality than for hemodialysis. When residual renal function lost, may be inadequate therapy.	Treatment by default. Often complicated by inattention to progressive cardiac and peripheral vascular disease. Long-term amyloidosis, malnutrition, depression.	All kidney-transplant programs preselect those patients with fewest complications. Exclusion of those older than 50 for pancreas + kidney simultaneous grafting obviously favorably prejudices outcome.
Relative cost	Has been used to circumvent initial outlay for dialysis equipment required by hemodialysis. Expense of dialysate is about the same as a kidney transplant.	Less expensive than kidney transplant in first year; subsequent years most expensive due to professional fees and cost of supplies.	Pancreas + kidney engraftment most expensive. After first year, kidney transplant—alone—lowest cost option.

How does a kidney transplant help?

Successful kidney transplantation is an immediate cure for ESRD. The kidney is donated by a relative, unrelated friend, or a dead person (cadaver). It is difficult to compare kidney-transplant patients with dialysis patients in terms of how long they live or how well they do, because people selected for a transplant must generally be in pretty good health. Nevertheless, the complete renewal of life activities by the most successful transplant recipients is an impressive example of the best in modern medicine. In fact, some of the most stable transplant recipients have even had successful pregnancies.

Are there drawbacks to having a transplant?

The most serious drawback to transplant surgery is the toxic drugs that transplant recipients must take for the rest of their lives to prevent their bodies from rejecting the donated organ. The body's immune system identifies the foreign kidney as an invader and tries to get rid of it. Immunosuppressant drugs turn off the immune system and allow the transplanted kidney to do its work. Ironically, these drugs are also strong enough to be damaging to the kidney.

More than 90% of people who get a kidney transplant survive the first year, compared to 80% on dialysis. About one in five transplant patients survive into the second decade (more than 10 years). A kidney transplant is highly preferred for newly diagnosed people with diabetes and ESRD under the age of 60.

Can a pancreas transplant cure diabetes?

Yes, pancreas and islet transplants are the only treatments that can "cure" type 1 diabetes. A cure means that you no longer have to inject insulin or balance food, exercise, and insulin as long as the transplant works. For ESRD patients with type 1 diabetes, combining a pancreas transplant with a kidney transplant is now routine at most U.S. hospitals. If you are scheduled for a kidney transplant, check with your doctor about getting a pancreas as well. If it is not offered at your hospital, you may want to locate a center that does. Pancreas-kidney recipients are not only dialysis free but also insulin free. The pancreas usually comes from a cadaver and the kidney from a living donor. It is also possible to transplant one kidney and half of a pancreas from a living donor.

In one remarkable series of 995 patients with diabetes, function of both organs one year after the transplant was 84%. More than 90% of pancreas-kidney recipients in a worldwide registry were alive at one year, more than 80% had functioning kidney grafts, and more than 70% no longer required insulin. Whether having normal blood glucose levels from the pancreas transplant will stop the progression of diabetic vascular complications is now a major research question. The increasingly better prognosis for people with diabetic kidney disease shows that we are making steady progress against this disease.

What about pancreas transplants alone for people with diabetes?

These might be considered for people with brittle diabetes who have hypoglycemia unawareness, but again, no one knows how they'll respond to immunosuppressant drugs.

At this point, only 5% of pancreas transplants are single transplants. This may change because there are new drugs—tacrolimus (Prograf) and mycophenolate mofetil (CellCept)—to supplement or replace cyclosporine that have resulted in a very low rejection rate. Indeed, the combination of these three drugs has allowed many patients to be withdrawn from the cortisone steroid-type of drugs that have been a mainstay of antirejection treatment but have side effects involving the bones and skin. This improvement in immunosuppression may lead to more single pancreas transplants in the next few years.

A renewed interest in human islet transplants has followed reports of the success of islet cell transplants done at the University of Edmonton using newer immune technologies.

Are transplanted islet cells an option?

Researchers in the area of islet transplantation believe the answer is yes. As early as 1989, studies proved that transplanted islets could make insulin and result in normal blood sugars. However, not much progress was made during the next 10 years. With recent success, the number of islet transplant research studies is growing once again.

Where do we get islets for transplantation?

Islets are obtained from the pancreas of someone who has died. Donors or their relatives have given permission to use their organs for transplantation and research. Great care is used to select a healthy pancreas for an islet transplant. Special solutions and procedures are used to free the islet cells, which can only be seen under a microscope, from the donor pancreas. The processing of the islets takes about 6 to 8 hours. In some studies, it took about 10,000 islet equivalents (IE) per kilogram of body weight for each patient to be free from insulin injections for a limited time. That would be approximately 700,000 islets for a person weighing 154 pounds. It takes 2–4 pancreases to get that many islets.

Can a living family member or friend donate islets?

Frequently, a family member will offer to donate islets to someone with diabetes. Although attempts have been made in the past to transplant islets from a living donor, the islets are obtained by taking part of the donor's pancreas, and the number of islets from a partial pancreas is not enough to get a patient free of insulin shots. Secondly, with removal of part of the pancreas, the donor may have a greater risk for developing diabetes later in life.

What is happening in islet research now?

Researchers report success in getting several people off insulin shots for a limited time through islet transplantation. The "Edmonton Protocol" is a research study that uses antirejection drugs without steroids and gives separate islet transplants over a one- to two-month period. Of the first 7 patients receiving this experimental treatment, all were able to be free of insulin shots for a prolonged period. As a result, multicenter clinical research trials have begun in the area of islet transplantation for the first time in history. These studies are sponsored by the Immune Tolerance Network (ITN) and are funded through the National Institutes of Health (NIH). Other centers are doing islet transplant research as well. The results of these studies will help determine whether islet transplantation can become a future treatment of choice for type 1 diabetes. Other researchers are working on encapsulating (coating) islets to eliminate the need for anti-rejection drugs.

How are islets transplanted?

An islet transplant is done under local anesthesia. A small area of skin on the abdomen is injected with a medicine to numb the area during the procedure. A radiologist injects the islets through a small tube into the liver, where they are nourished by the liver's blood supply. The islets start making insulin immediately when transplanted. If conditions are right, the islets will attach in the liver and continue making insulin in response to blood sugar levels in the body. Most patients are in the hospital only 1 to 3 days.

What happens after an islet transplant?

Each patient is followed closely, with frequent blood tests and doctor visits to check how well the islets are working and to see if there are any side effects from the transplant or the medications. Patients have to check blood sugar several times a day to see how the islets are working and visit the study doctors for periodic tests.

Most of the centers doing islet research will have research money to pay for the cost of the antirejection medications for about a year, but patients (and perhaps health insurance companies) will need to cover the high costs of the medications afterward. People interested in getting an islet transplant should talk with the study doctors and with their health insurance company about whether any financial help is available.

Islet transplantation does have significant risks, which should be listed in detail on the consent form for each study. Each person considering an islet transplant should read the consent form carefully. The benefits and risks should be discussed with the study doctors and with the primary care physician and health care team.

Will islet transplantation cure diabetes?

In the first 17 patients in the Edmonton study, some patients had to go back on insulin, so the longest successful transplant is still just over 5 years. Researchers do not know if the newer procedures and antirejection medications will increase how long islets will work.

Is an artificial pancreas an option?

It may be possible to have an artificial pancreas implanted sometime soon, just as pumps are implanted now. All that is lacking is a way to measure blood glucose levels consistently. Once this meter is invented, you might have an artificial pancreas and no need for immunosuppressant drugs.

How successful are organ transplants?

The United Network for Organ Sharing (UNOS) maintains an organ registry, and the outcome of nearly every surgery is known. For patients who received a pancreas-kidney transplant, 85% were dialysis free at 1 year, and 80% at 3 years.

These dialysis-free rates were higher than for patients with diabetes who received only a kidney transplant. The pancreas, although it may require additional surgery, helps the transplanted kidney do its work. The rejection rate at 1 year for a pancreas-kidney transplant is only 3% and for the pancreas alone is less than 10%. Thus, most recipients of a successful transplant can expect to remain insulin free for years or for the rest of their lives.

What are the side effects of immunosuppressant drugs?

Both tacrolimus and cyclosporine can decrease kidney function, which can be a problem for people who already have kidney damage from diabetes. In those who have good kidney function, both tacrolimus and cyclosporine are usually well tolerated, but other side effects of the immunosuppressant drugs also occur, including a tendency toward obesity or osteoporosis with the cortisone-like drugs. Again, cortisone-like drugs are not being used as much, especially with the introduction of Prograf and CellCept. However, at this time, you have no choice but to take some immunosuppressant drug after the transplant. The side effects must be accepted as a trade-off for being insulin free and must be considered before the surgery. Ironically, some type 1 patients who receive a transplant develop type 2 diabetes due to drug toxicity from their immunosuppressive drugs.

Who usually gets a transplant?

The typical candidate for a pancreas-kidney transplant has had diabetes for 15–30 years, has developed high blood pressure, and has had an increase in blood levels of creatinine associated with kidney failure. At this point, the nephrologist should consult with the transplant surgeon and either arrange for the patient to go on the waiting list for a donor kidney transplant or screen family members to determine who is suitable to be a kidney or kidney and half-pancreas donor. The organs that come from a living relative are more likely to be accepted by the patient's body.

The timing of when to do the kidney transplant depends on both creatinine blood levels and the patient's symptoms. Chronic fatigue and a need for blood pressure medications, along with recurrent swelling or need for diuretic (water) pills, indicate that the individual will eventually need dialysis. At this point, the patient should be placed on the waiting list or a living-donor transplant should be arranged.

Will more transplants be done for people with diabetes in the future?

It seems likely. The recipient of a successful transplant is restored to health. Add to that the increasing availability of organs for transplant and the fact that the cost of a transplant when spread over the years of good health afterward is not as expensive as the dialysis option. The results of ongoing research into new and better drugs or techniques to suppress the immune system will lead to transplants being an even more popular option for people with diabetes.

Eli A. Friedman, MD; David E.R. Sutherland, MD, PhD; and Karen Flavin, RN, CCRC, contributed to this chapter.

10

Peripheral Vascular Disease

Case study

HG is a 54-year-old contractor who has had diabetes for 15 years and maintains irregular control. He is overweight, and his only regular exercise is manual labor as a contractor. HG smoked one pack of cigarettes a day for 20 years, until he quit 2 years ago after a severe respiratory illness.

HG has developed an ulcer on his foot that would not heal, despite two courses of antibiotics. An evaluation revealed that HG had pulses that could be felt in the groin (femoral pulses) and in the knee (popliteal pulses) but no foot pulses. Circulation tests using a Doppler device revealed a moderately poor blood supply to the foot. For 5 years, HG had noticed increasing pain in the left calf after walking shorter and shorter distances. Although this was not disabling and did not interfere with his work, HG was perplexed because his right leg seemed fine. HG also complained of numbness, tingling, and hot and cold sensations in both feet. He felt these were caused by poor circulation and used various heat remedies during and after work.

His doctor pointed out the diminished hair and thinning of the skin on the left foot compared with the right. Doppler signals were much stronger in the right foot. To encourage healing of the ulcer, he was referred to a vascular surgeon who ordered a magnetic resonance angioscopy (MRA) to view the blood vessels in his feet and legs.

The MRA revealed that the femoral artery (groin) and popliteal arteries (knee) had impared circulation (Figure 10-1). There was complete blockage of the arteries below the knee (anterior tibial and posterior tibial, with severe disease of the peroneal artery). However, the dorsalis pedis artery in the foot was not badly impaired; HG had good blood vessels in his feet.

At a family meeting, the surgeon described a bypass operation that would restore circulation from the good popliteal artery at the knee to the dorsalis pedis artery in the top of the foot. This would speed healing and save HG's toe.

What puts you at risk of developing peripheral vascular disease?

Peripheral vascular disease (PVD) is a condition in which plaque buildup causes a narrowing of the arteries to your legs. The case study is a typical example of PVD in patients with diabetes. PVD is 20 times more common in people with diabetes than in the general population. Other risk factors are smoking, lack of exercise, high blood pressure, high blood lipid levels (including cholesterol), and obesity. Women with diabetes are just as much at risk, and the disease is not limited to the elderly. It depends on genetics and how long you have had diabetes. It is a serious disease that needs to be recognized and treated.

How is the diagnosis of PVD different for people with diabetes?

People with diabetes are more likely to have atherosclerosis involving the arteries between the knee and the foot. It is not enough for your physician to check for adequate circulation by feeling a popliteal pulse (Figure 10-1).

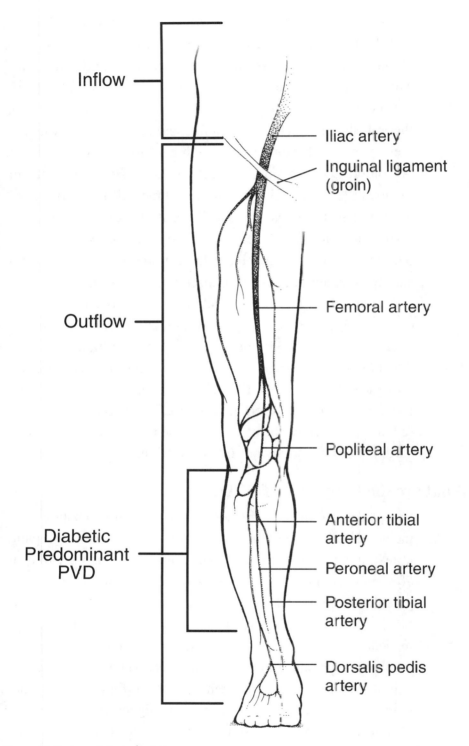

Figure 10-1. Leg arteries and veins.

A major difference in the arteries of people with diabetes is that the arterial walls frequently contain extensive calcium (Mönckeberg's sclerosis), making the arteries rigid and hard. This is associated with nerve damage (neuropathy). They are not blocked, but the physician will be unable to feel a pulse in them. If the physician checks ankle and arm blood pressures, these pressures become falsely high because the vessels cannot be compressed to be measured. So higher systolic pressures in the lower leg or a high ankle-to-arm (brachial) ratio does not guarantee that there is adequate circulation. An alternative to taking ankle-arm pressures is to measure toe pressures, because they do not have the calcification problem, or to measure the oxygen in the skin (transcutaneous) of the feet.

Studies show that poor circulation was associated with 62% of cases of nonhealing ulceration and was a cause in 46% of amputations. Remember that adequate blood flow to the skin not only depends on the arteries but may be greatly influenced by other factors, including skin integrity, death of tissue (necrosis) from repeated trauma, tissue swelling (edema), congestive heart failure or heart conditions with low cardiac output, and uncontrolled infection.

What are the symptoms of PVD?

Symptoms that indicate the need for a vascular evaluation include claudication (pain in the calves while exercising); pain at rest; night pain; and ulceration, gangrene, or inability to heal after minor foot surgery. Claudication is the inability to walk a given distance, usually stated in the number of city blocks (one block = 75 yards), because of muscle pain or cramping due to inadequate blood supply. The location of the muscle groups involved helps your physician distinguish whether the blockage is in the arteries (inflow) or veins (outflow) (Figure 10-1). The higher up the involved muscles are, the higher the blockage is. Claudication is made worse by an incline or a faster pace, and it is almost always relieved by rest. PVD must also be distinguished from nerve irritation such as arthritis, a herniated disk, tarsal tunnel syndrome, or neuropathy itself. In the case study, HG's claudication was an early sign of insufficient blood flow in the affected leg. He also had neuropathy.

Intermittent claudication does not mean you are going to lose the limb, especially in its early stages. Only 10–15% of patients go on to more limb-threatening symptoms. Some patients with diabetes, especially those who smoke, may progress more rapidly. Progressive claudication with walking less than 1/2 to 1 city block or that interferes with your lifestyle or work indicates a need for a vascular consultation and treatment. Limb-threatening symptoms include pain at rest and tissue loss. Patients with impaired circulation to their legs and feet tend to describe a deep, aching pain in the foot, which feels better with support of the area.

How is PVD diagnosed?

The physician must assess poor circulation in your legs and feet. In population-based studies, 20–30% of patients had absent foot pulses. Also, hair growth, skin and nail texture, pallor of the foot when elevated, redness of the foot when it hangs down, and the appearance and temperature of the affected foot compared with the other foot are important to consider. There are no laboratory tests that will always measure the degree of poor circulation or predict healing. This includes Doppler pressures, ankle-arm blood pressure ratios, toe pressures, waveform analyses, pulse-volume recordings, laser Doppler, transcutaneous (skin) oxygen determination, and MRA. Arteriography (dye studies of the arteries) is indicated when there are ulcers or wounds that fail to heal and areas that repeatedly break down despite therapeutic shoes.

Blood flow can be checked by feeling arterial pulses in the feet and legs. When pulses are diminished or absent, noninvasive Doppler arterial testing is performed to determine the differences in blood pressures from the foot to the thigh.

Pressures can be compared to the opposite side and to the arm to locate potential sites of arterial blockage in the leg.

How does the doctor decide what to do?

PVD can be studied with the use of arteriograms or MRAs as necessary. Bypass surgery may be done to improve the blood flow through the arteries to the feet. With the help of arteriograms, more than 90% of patients with diabetes who have ischemic foot lesions (blockages in the arteries of the foot) can have the blockages surgically corrected. MRA may replace arteriography as the procedure of choice to visualize blood vessels in the leg down to and into the foot. Otherwise, because of the increased incidence of dye-related kidney complications, your physician must prepare you carefully and give you intravenous fluids before and after the angiogram. Theophylline and aminophylline alone or in combination will decrease the likelihood of dye-related kidney problems.

You may be a candidate for bypass, depending on your other risk factors and overall well-being. Elderly patients who have severe dementia or mental deterioration and do not walk are not candidates for bypass surgery. Patients with extensive tissue damage or who would probably lose the limb even if the circulation were restored must be carefully evaluated as to whether they would be better served by amputation. Age by itself is not a reason not to have vascular surgery. Cost is also not a problem, because an aggressive approach to saving a limb is cost-effective. It is important for you and your health care team to assess your risk factors and other health conditions that might affect the outcome.

What needs to be done before you have bypass surgery?

Coronary artery disease is the leading cause of complications and death in all major vascular procedures. That is why it is so important for your heart health to be evaluated and treated before the operation (chapter 5). Active infection must be controlled before any surgery. Intravenous antibiotics are needed. The choice of anesthesia is basically up to you and your team because all have been found equally safe.

What techniques might the physician use to restore inflow circulation?

The treatment used to correct blood vessel blockages depends on the location and extent of the blockage and your other risk factors and general health. Your physician must be experienced with patients with diabetes and have a flexible approach. He or she will choose among the following procedures: endarterectomy, bypass grafting, angioplasty and laser surgery, and balloon angioplasty.

Endarterectomy

Endarterectomy is a "cleaning out" of the diseased artery. It was one of the earliest treatments but has been largely replaced by bypass grafting or balloon angioplasty. Local endarterectomy is still the procedure of choice for treatment of carotid artery disease.

Angioplasty and laser therapy

Endovascular (inside the blood vessel) techniques have been made possible by advances in technology, plastics, and optics. Space-age technology includes percutaneous transluminal angioplasty (PTA), atherectomy (rotarblade), and lasers to clear out the blood vessels. Almost all of the currently used endovascular techniques require balloon angioplasty to open the vessel wide enough for adequate blood flow. A balloon angioplasty is a procedure in which a balloon attached to a catheter (tube) is inserted into the narrowed part of the blood vessel. The balloon is then expanded to widen this part of the artery. In some cases, the surgeon will also use a stent, a tiny metal device shaped like a spring or mesh cylinder that is inserted with the balloon, expanded, and left in the blood vessel to hold it open.

It is important to understand that differences in success of endovascular procedures are based on *1*) the location of the blockage or narrowing, *2*) length of the blockage or narrowing, *3*) localized versus widespread narrowing or blockage, and *4*) composition of the plaque (calcium). Most suitable for endovascular techniques are short narrowings in arteries that are otherwise disease free. The iliac arteries (supplying blood to the lower body and legs) lend themselves to the best results, with overall initial and long-term success rates equal to those of surgery. Narrowing or blockage farther down in the lower leg or longer blockages, more widespread disease, heavily calcified plaques, and total blockage lead to less successful endovascular techniques. However, these are typical conditions in a person with diabetes and have to be evaluated. Endovascular procedures often go along with surgery when they can restore inflow and a bypass can restore circulation to a lower-leg blockage. Again a team approach helps ensure success.

What techniques might the physician use to restore outflow circulation?

Procedures to restore circulation in the lower leg require the use of a vein to put in place to provide a path for blood to flow around the blockage. The saphenous vein in the leg is the one most frequently used. Synthetic grafts don't work as well. People with diabetes and extensive tissue loss or gangrene of the foot need to have restoration of a pulse to the foot whenever possible for the most rapid and effective healing. Bypasses can be done all the way down to the foot arteries (Figure 10-1) and their branches to achieve this. Bypasses on legs and feet are complex and challenging procedures and are only considered when there is limb-threatening ischemia. Even

5 years after surgery, these bypass surgeries have successfully saved the limb in 87–92% of cases. You may also be asked to take certain drugs, such as aspirin or Trendral to encourage better circulation.

What are the drawbacks of bypass surgery?

Complication rates associated with surgery are similar to those in patients with diabetes who undergo major amputation alone, so why not take an aggressive approach to saving the leg and foot? Bypass surgery is often your best option because the endovascular procedures (done inside the artery) have limited success and a very high complication rate because of the nature of diabetic lower-leg atherosclerosis.

This chapter was written by Gary W. Gibbons, MD, and Sheilah A. Janus.

11

Peripheral Neuropathy

Case study

Mrs. Johnson is 52 years old and has had type 2 diabetes for 20 years. Recently her feet began to burn. She was just diagnosed with painful neuropathy in her feet. Her doctor checked the reflexes at her ankles and knees. He also checked her feet with a tuning fork and a thin wire called a monofilament, and found that Mrs. Johnson had lost some sensation in her feet. This meant that she was at risk of injuring her foot and not realizing it, which could lead to a foot ulcer.

Introduction

Peripheral neuropathy (nerve damage) is the most common long-term complication of diabetes. It affects as many as 75% of all people with diabetes. The symptoms of neuropathy range from unpleasant to severe. On average, the symptoms occur within 10 years after the onset of diabetes. Unfortunately, for many people with type 2 diabetes, the symptoms of neuropathy may be the first sign of the diabetes that they have actually had for many years. You may develop painful neuropathy soon after you begin treating your diabetes with insulin or a sulfonylurea. As your blood glucose levels improve, the pain should go away, but the symptoms may last for as long as 6–18 months. Be patient; improving blood sugar makes your whole body healthier.

Peripheral neuropathy is also called sensorimotor neuropathy. It usually happens in both limbs at once; and when people with diabetes say they have neuropathy, this is usually what they mean. Table 11-1 outlines the symptoms that can occur.

What is peripheral neuropathy?

Neuropathy is damage to the nerves. Nerves connect your brain to your spinal cord, your organs, and other parts of your body. This is called your nervous system and has several parts—the central nervous system, the peripheral nervous system, and the autonomic nervous system. The central nervous system is made up of the brain and the spinal cord. The peripheral nervous system is made up of the nerves that go farther out to areas such as your feet and toes. Because most nerve damage from diabetes occurs in the peripheral nervous system, it is called peripheral neuropathy. This type of neuropathy affects the sensory nerves, with damage to the longer

Table 11-1. Peripheral Neuropathy and Its Symptoms

Syndrome	Symptoms
Small-fiber damage	• Loss of ability to detect temperature • "Pins and needles," tingling or burning sensation • Pain, usually worse at night • Numbness or loss of feeling • Cold extremities • Swelling of feet
Large-fiber damage	• Abnormal or unusual sensations • Loss of balance • Inability to sense position of toes and feet • Charcot's joint
Motor nerve damage	• Loss of muscle tone in hands and feet • Misshapen or deformed toes and feet • Callus formation • Open sores or ulcers on feet

nerves first. That is why the symptoms begin in the feet, and sometimes the hands, and move up. It is also called "stocking-glove" syndrome because of where the symptoms occur.

The sensorimotor nervous system includes your sensory and motor nerves. The sensory nerves send information about how things feel from the skin and internal organs to the brain. The motor nerves send information about movement from the brain to the body. For example, if you step on a sharp tack with your bare foot, the sensory nerves send a message to your brain that you are in pain. The brain then sends a message back to the motor nerves telling your foot to move off the tack.

The autonomic nervous system controls involuntary or automatic functions, such as heart rate, digestion, and bladder and sexual function. For example, the autonomic nervous system tells your heart to speed up when you are running and slow down when you stop. It helps maintain your blood pressure whether you are standing, sitting, or lying down.

What causes peripheral neuropathy?

Neuropathy can occur from a variety of chronic illnesses such as diabetes or cancer or from exposure to toxins such as alcohol, heavy metals, or chemotherapy drugs. The causes of neuropathy are not completely known, but in diabetes, it is related to high blood glucose over a long period. The DCCT showed that intensive insulin therapy lowered the risk for neuropathy by 60% for participants in that study, who all had type 1 diabetes. The Japanese (Kumamoto) study and the UKPDS of people with type 2 diabetes show the same beneficial effects of good blood glucose control. For people with type 2 diabetes, high blood glucose, decreased insulin output by the pancreas, age, obesity, and duration of diabetes have all been linked to neuropathy. It is probably fair to say that neuropathy is caused not only by elevated blood glucose levels but also by a combination of genetic influences and environmental factors.

How do high blood glucose levels cause nerve damage?

There are several theories about why neuropathy occurs when blood glucose levels are high for a long period. Unlike most cells in the body, nerve cells don't need insulin to pull in glucose from the bloodstream. Therefore, when blood glucose levels are above normal, the glucose level inside the nerve cells is also high. These high glucose levels may be toxic to the nerves.

Inside the cell, glucose is broken down into a substance called *sorbitol* (a sugar alcohol) by an enzyme called *aldose reductase*. Sorbitol is then converted to a form of sugar called *fructose* by another enzyme. In people with diabetes, the levels of glucose, sorbitol, and fructose are all high, which may damage nerves. One class of drugs being tested for the treatment of diabetic neuropathy is *aldose reductase inhibitors* (ARIs). ARIs prevent the breakdown of glucose into sorbitol in the nerve cells.

The reasons that elevated sorbitol and sugar levels damage nerves may be related to decreased *myo*-inositol levels, a substance that your nerves need to function normally. Glucose and *myo*-inositol molecules have similar sizes and shapes, and they compete to get into the cells. Glucose wins over *myo*-inositol, so when glucose levels are higher inside the cells, *myo*-inositol levels are lower. The cells are not able to function normally without adequate *myo*-inositol.

Another theory to account for nerve damage is glycation (sugar coating) of proteins in the nerve cells. When glucose levels are high, glucose molecules stick to the protein molecules that make up new cells. (This is similar to the way glucose builds up on the red blood cells and is measured with an A1C test.) This buildup prevents the nerve cells from working normally. Their ability to send and receive signals from the brain and spinal cord may be impaired.

Another theory is based on the decreased blood flow that can occur when small blood vessels are damaged from diabetes. Decreased blood flow to the peripheral nerves may damage them over time.

People with type 1 diabetes have trouble converting some of the building blocks of fatty acids into the fatty acids that are necessary for the cells to function. As a result, there is an inadequate amount of some of the fatty acids that the cell needs.

Autoimmunity has also been suggested as a reason for nerve damage. The damaged nerves may be misread as germs and the antibodies that develop are directed toward the nerves.

What are the symptoms of neuropathy?

You can have problems with nerve damage without having any symptoms, so you and your doctor may be unaware of the neuropathy. The most common symptoms are pain, tingling, or burning in the feet and legs or numbness of the feet. The symptoms depend on the nerves affected and the extent of the damage. Sometimes, numbness is the only sign. Diabetes can cause damage to the autonomic, sensory, and motor nerves. (See chapters 5, 12, 13, 17 and 18.)

How is neuropathy diagnosed?

Neuropathy can be diagnosed by the symptoms. At least once a year, your health care provider should test your reflexes and check your bare feet for their ability to sense heat and cold, vibrations with a tuning fork, and a light touch with a monofilament (plastic wire).

Why is neuropathy so serious?

When sensory nerves are damaged, you cannot feel heat, cold, or pain. Because there is no pain, you may continue to walk on an injured foot. This can result in an ulcer, which can become infected, leading to gangrene and amputation. Because there is loss of feeling, you must check your feet every day or have a family member do it for you (chapter 3). Ask your provider or nurse educator to show you the proper way to inspect your feet and how to care for them. If you need help, do not be embarrassed to say so.

Nerves are made up of both small and large fibers. If the small fibers of the nerves are affected, you will have pain and be unable to detect heat and cold, which increases your risk for burns or frostbite. If large fibers are affected, you lose the ability to sense the position of your feet or to feel a light touch.

If the pain that results from sensorimotor neuropathy lasts for less than 6 months, it is considered acute. Pain that lasts longer than 6 months is considered chronic. With chronic painful neuropathy, the pain may eventually disappear, and your feet and hands will feel numb or always cold as the nerves become more damaged.

With large-fiber damage, your senses of balance and position are impaired, which increases your risk for falls. Some people describe this as "not being able to feel where my feet are when I walk." These people have extra difficulty walking in the dark.

When motor nerves are damaged, the muscles in the feet can become weak and eventually atrophy (degenerate). This results in the development of foot and toe deformities, such as hammertoes and claw toes.

What if your only symptom is numbness?

Actually, feet that feel numb are more common than painful feet. If you are unable to feel a tuning fork that is vibrating on your toe or a wire pressing on the fleshy part of your foot, you have an insensate foot, like Mrs. Johnson in the case study. If you have any foot deformity, you can protect your feet with custom-made orthotics or shoes. These can save your feet. See chapter 3 for information on shoes and foot care.

What is the treatment for neuropathy?

The treatment for peripheral neuropathy is based on the symptoms you have. There is no cure for neuropathy, so the treatment is mostly aimed at relieving the pain and protecting your feet and hands to prevent injuries. Lowering blood glucose levels as near normal as possible may decrease pain or other symptoms. Things you can do to care for neuropathy are listed in Table 11-2.

There are medicines that can be used to relieve pain and other symptoms. Vitamins alone usually aren't effective to treat neuropathy caused by diabetes. Pain-relieving medicines that contain narcotics are generally not recommended because of side effects and the risk for addiction. Over-the-counter pain relievers and topical capsaicin 0.075% (Zostrix HP) cream applied to the skin may be effective for burning pain. Medicines that your provider may prescribe include low doses of anticonvulsive agents and antidepressants. Many of these medicines take time to work, so you need to give them a fair trial (4–6 weeks) before you decide whether they are effective. Like all medicines, these may cause side effects. Common ones are sleepiness, dry mouth, constipation, nausea, memory problems, and dizziness. Taking your dose at bedtime may help. Tell your provider about these or any other side effects. Your dose may need to be adjusted. Obviously, there are many drugs to choose from, and they need to be discussed with your doctor. Sometimes, it may be helpful to see a neurologist.

Therapies used in place of or along with medications can also be helpful. Walking or gentle stretching, relaxation exercises, biofeedback, and hypnosis may help relieve your pain. Stopping alcohol drinking and cigarette smoking may help relieve symptoms. Elastic body stockings (available at dance or exercise stores), pantyhose, or foot cradles can help keep clothes and bedcovers away from your sensitive skin. Lamb's

Table 11-2. Self-care Practices for Peripheral Neuropathy

- Keep your blood sugar levels as close to normal as is safe for you.

- Protect your feet. You need to do what your nerves used to do for you. (See chapter 3 about foot care.)

- Give therapies a fair trial before you decide whether they are working. Some medicines take time before they begin to work.

- Talk to your provider about any "home" or other remedies you are using or hear about. Some may be helpful, but others may actually be harmful.

- Stop cigarette smoking. Ask your provider about smoking cessation programs. Nicotine delivery systems (patches, gum) are available without a prescription and may help you quit.

- Avoid alcohol because it can increase nerve damage. Ask your provider about programs that can help if you believe alcohol is a problem for you.

- Keep informed and up-to-date. Take diabetes education classes to learn the best and latest techniques for protecting your health. Neuropathy is an area of ongoing research. Ask your provider periodically if there are new medicines or other therapies available. If you are interested in participating in studies of new medications, call the ADA at 1-800-DIABETES, look up diabetes or diabetic neuropathy on the Internet, or contact the diabetes program offered at large medical centers in your area and ask if there are any studies available.

wool padding and specially made shoes or orthotic devices can help protect misshapen feet.

Transcutaneous nerve stimulation (TENS) units are battery-operated devices that are about the size of a portable radio. TENS units provide small electrical impulses that block the pain message from getting to your brain. These devices are available only by prescription. There are also clinics in larger medical centers that specialize in pain relief. Ask your provider for a referral if you believe this would be helpful to you. Talk to your physician or nurse educator about any pain remedies you read about in newspapers or magazines. Many of these are expensive but not very effective.

Are there treatments for the pain of neuropathy?

Try simple maneuvers first. Painful neuropathy can actually be brought on by beginning to improve BG levels; but it usually goes away as you maintain near normal BG levels. It may take as long as 6 to 18 months.

Capsaicin

Burning pain may respond to capsaicin cream applied three or four times daily. Capsaicin is extracted from chili peppers. Take care to avoid eyes and genitals, and wear gloves when applying the cream. It is safer to cover the affected areas with plastic wrap. Initially the symptoms may get worse, followed by relief of pain in 2–3 weeks.

Nerve blocking

Lidocaine given by slow infusion has provided relief of pain for 3–21 days. This form of therapy may be most useful in self-limited forms of neuropathy. If successful, therapy can be continued with oral mexiletine. These compounds target pain caused by sensitivity of nerve endings near the surface of the skin.

Antidepressants

Several studies have shown the tricyclic antidepressants given along with tranquilizers, such as phenothiazine or fluphenazine, to be effective in treating painful neuropathy. These drugs act by interrupting pain transmission. Talk with your doctor about how these drugs may increase your risk of heart attack.

Gabapentin

Gabapentin (Neurontin) is an effective anticonvulsant that has been shown to relieve painful neuropathy. Topiramide may be an effective alternative.

Transcutaneous nerve stimulation

TENS may occasionally be helpful and certainly represents one of the more benign therapies for painful neuropathy. Move the electrodes around to identify sensitive areas and obtain the most relief.

Analgesics

These are rarely of much benefit in the treatment of painful neuropathy, although they may be of some use on a short-term basis.

Biofeedback, exercise, and support

Biofeedback programs help quite a bit, especially long-term, as does yoga because you learn more about your body. Exercise such as swimming or stationary bike riding releases natural pain relievers and improves BG levels. Find a knowledgeable health care team, which may include physicians who are experts in diabetes, endocrinology, and/or neurology; nurse educators; a dietitian; and a psychologist or social worker. Support groups and educational programs are often helpful. There is help available for you now and hope for the future as research seeks and finds new therapies.

This chapter was written by Martha M. Funnell, MS, RN, CDE; Douglas A. Greene, MD; Eva L. Feldman, MD, PhD; and Martin J. Stevens, MD. Aaron Vinik, MD, PhD, FCP, FACP, contributed to this chapter.

12

Autonomic Neuropathies

Introduction

Autonomic nerves help with the activities of your body that you don't have to think about—heartbeat, breathing, food digestion, etc. Neuropathy can further be classified as either diffuse or focal—*diffuse* meaning scattered and *focal* meaning only one or a few nerves are involved. Diffuse neuropathies develop slowly over time, and focal nerve damage tends to occur suddenly.

Damage to the autonomic nerves can affect major systems in your body, such as the heart (chapter 5), the stomach and intestines (chapter 13), or the sexual organs (chapters 17 and 18). This chapter deals with autonomic neuropathy in nerves affecting the bladder, eye, heart, sweat glands, and hypoglycemia awareness.

What are the possible causes of neuropathy?

There can be many causes of neuropathy. Diabetes is not the only one. To rule out the other possible causes, your provider must consider the family history of neuropathy, vitamin B-12 and folate deficiency, syphilis, Lyme disease, leprosy, autoimmune diseases, and toxic causes of neuropathy including alcoholism, arsenic, and a variety of drugs. Tests to confirm or rule out these other conditions will need to be done. The condition causing your neuropathy must be treated along with the neuropathy if you are to get well.

How is diabetic neuropathy diagnosed?

To diagnose neuropathy, your health care provider may gather information from five different categories. First, of course, are your symptoms (Table 12-1). For autonomic neuropathy, it is necessary to check your body's responses to stimuli, for example, in the heart or gastrointestinal wall. There is a series of simple, noninvasive tests for detecting cardiovascular autonomic neuropathy. These tests are based on detection of heart rate and blood pressure response to a series of physical maneuvers. Specific tests are used to evaluate gastrointestinal, genitourinary, sweating function, and peripheral skin blood flow, all of which can be affected by autonomic diabetic neuropathy.

How does autonomic neuropathy affect your bladder?

The genitourinary system includes both bladder and sex organs. The kidneys filter your blood and make urine to take away waste products. The urine goes from the kidney through the ureter into the bladder. The bladder is elastic and can expand and contract. After about 1 1/2 cups (10 oz) of urine collects in your bladder, you feel the urge to go to the bathroom. Bladder function is controlled by three different types of nerves. One transmits the signal to your brain when your bladder is full. Another causes your bladder to contract so you can pass urine. A third maintains the tone of the sphincter that opens for you to urinate and closes when you are finished. Diabetes can cause damage to all three types of nerves.

What are the symptoms of neuropathy of the bladder?

When people first begin to have this type of damage, they may urinate less often. Some people will have urgency and frequency but will pass only small amounts of urine each time.

Table 12-1. Symptoms of Diabetic Autonomic Neuropathies

Classification	Symptoms
Genitourinary	
Bladder	• Urinating less often • Frequent urinary tract infections • Difficulty emptying bladder completely • Weak urinary stream • Difficulty starting to urinate and dribbling afterwards; incontinence
Sexual function	*In males:* • Impotence *In females:* • Diminished vaginal lubrication • Decreased frequency of orgasm
Gastrointestinal	
Stomach	• Difficulty swallowing • Feeling full just after beginning to eat • Bloating and abdominal pain • Hypoglycemia after meals • Nausea without vomiting • Vomiting food that was eaten many hours before
Intestinal	• Diarrhea, especially at night • Constipation
Cardiovascular	• Swelling in feet • Severe dizziness on standing • Fixed heart rate • Short of breath on exertion
Counterregulation	• Loss of early warning symptoms of hypoglycemia
Sweating	• Dry hands and feet • Increased sweating on upper body • Sweating while eating certain foods
Pupils	• Delayed or absent response of pupils to darkness/light • Decreased pupil size

This is because the bladder does not empty completely each time. Tests for bladder function might include blood tests of your kidney function, measurement of the amount of urine left in your bladder after you urinate, or an ultrasound test of your bladder when it is full.

One of the concerns is that urine remaining in your bladder provides an excellent medium for bacteria to grow, especially if there is also glucose in the urine. This can cause a bladder or urinary tract infection (UTI). If untreated, these infections can cause kidney damage. Symptoms of a bladder infection are frequent urination of small amounts, pain or burning when you urinate, being unable to urinate even though you feel the urge, and dark-colored urine. UTIs usually go away quickly with antibiotics. You need to call your provider at the first signs of an infection. If you have more than two bladder infections each year, it may be an early sign of nerve damage to your bladder. If this is true for you, talk to your provider about the need for tests of your bladder function.

What is the treatment for bladder neuropathy?

The treatment for bladder dysfunction includes both self-care activities and drug therapies. Patients with neurogenic bladder may not feel when their bladders are full. You'll have to think for your bladder. Drink plenty of fluids and go to the bathroom every 2 hours. You may need to press on your bladder to determine when it is full, and if necessary, push on it to start the flow of urine. Medicines to improve bladder function are available and may be effective. Drugs such as bethanechol are sometimes helpful, but they often do not help you fully empty your bladder. The sphincter can be relaxed with terazosin or doxazosin. Self-catheterization can be useful in the case of a contracted sphincter, with generally a low risk of infection. Bladder neck surgery may help to relieve spasm of the internal sphincter. Because the external sphincter remains intact, urine will not leak out.

How does autonomic neuropathy affect your eyes?

The pupils in your eyes react to light and darkness by becoming smaller in very bright light and larger when it is dark. The response of the pupils is controlled by autonomic nerves. If these nerves are damaged, the pupils respond more slowly to darkness, so it can take longer for your eyes to adjust when you enter a dark room. You may have more difficulty driving at night because your eyes don't respond as quickly to the lights of an oncoming car or when going from a well-lit to a darker area. You need to take precautions to ensure your safety in these situations.

How does autonomic neuropathy affect your cardiovascular system?

Autonomic nerves control your heart rate and blood pressure, which normally change slightly throughout the day in response to position (lying, sitting, and standing), stress, exercise, breathing patterns, and sleep. If the nerves to the heart and blood vessels are damaged by diabetes, the blood pressure and heart rate may respond more slowly to these factors.

If the nerves that regulate your blood pressure are damaged, blood pressure can drop quickly when you stand up and not return to a normal level as quickly as it did before the nerves were damaged. You may feel lightheaded or dizzy, see black spots, or even pass out. This is called *orthostatic hypotension*. This results from blood pooling in the feet, which can lead to swelling or edema. Orthostatic hypotension is often a late development of autonomic neuropathy in patients with diabetes.

How is orthostatic hypotension diagnosed?

Because it is not unusual to feel lightheaded when you stand up too quickly, your provider needs to take your blood pressure and heart rate when you are lying and standing to diagnose orthostatic hypotension. This should be done at least once a year. If you have concerns, ask your provider to do these simple tests again.

The situation can be complicated by the fact that people with advanced diabetes may have complications involving the kidney, eyes, and blood vessels, making it difficult to determine which condition is responsible for the patient's symptoms. There is also "meal-induced hypotension," in which people become dizzy soon after breakfast, occasionally after lunch, but not at all with dinner. It is difficult to relieve the morning or breakfast-related low blood pressure without making the afternoon or evening blood pressure high. Loss of the daily rhythm of blood pressure control is the hallmark of autonomic neuropathy: blood pressure tends to rise at night and fall during the day. There is a risk of stroke. Low blood pressure medications are discussed below.

What is the treatment for orthostatic hypotension?

Trying to elevate blood pressure in the standing position must be balanced against making it too high in the lying position. Treatment for orthostatic or postural hypotension includes better blood glucose control, an adequate salt intake to be sure that you have a large enough volume of plasma in your bloodstream, avoidance of medications such as diuretics, and safety measures to prevent falls. Raising the head of your bed on blocks (to a 30-degree angle) is helpful, and putting on waist-high elastic stockings before you get up may help prevent your blood pressure from dropping. You should put them on while lying down and not remove them until you have returned to lying down. Clearly, they can be uncomfortable, especially in hot weather, which means that people don't like to use them. In severe cases, you may need a total body stocking or an Air Force antigravity suit.

Medications such as fludrocortisone (Florinef) may help to expand plasma volume. You must be on the alert for edema (swelling), because there is a risk of developing hypertension and congestive heart failure. Other drugs (for example, phenylephrine, ephedrine, Neo-Synephrine nasal spray, beta blockers, clonidine, octreotide, and Epogen) that work more directly on the blood vessels are used to treat orthostatic hypotension. A few patients may be helped with propranolol

(Inderal). Postural hypotension that occurs after eating may respond to therapy with octreotide (Sandostatin).

Does autonomic neuropathy affect your heart rate?

If the nerves that control heart rate are affected, the heart rate tends to be fast and does not change very much in response to breathing patterns, exercise, stress, or sleep.

How is neuropathy's effect on your heart rate diagnosed?

It can be diagnosed through measuring the changes in your pulse as you breathe deeply, during a Valsalva maneuver (done by bearing down as hard as you can), or before and after standing. An electrocardiogram (ECG) and specialized computer programs may be used to do this. This effect on the heart is a serious complication because it may increase your risk for irregular heartbeat and prevent you from feeling the pain or warning symptoms of a heart attack.

Sometimes the nerve damage prevents you from getting the usual cardiovascular benefits from aerobic exercise. If this is the case, ask your provider what kind of exercise you can do.

Cardiac stress testing should be done in people in whom there is any question of heart disease, whether there is pain or not. This is especially true if the person has two or more risk factors for coronary artery disease (see chapter 5).

How are changes in the daily pattern of blood pressures connected with the risk of sudden death?

Normally, blood pressure declines at night. It has been shown that people with type 1 and type 2 diabetes and albuminuria (protein in the urine) have blunted blood pressure cycles and that their hearts may be at full throttle all the time, which may help explain the cardiovascular events that occur in this high-risk group. Damage to the vagus nerve, which supplies the lungs and heart and regulates blood pressure, may be an important factor in sudden cardiovascular death and silent heart attacks. These findings help explain the mortality risk for people with autonomic failure. When you are taking blood pressure medication and you have blunted or reversed blood pressure patterns, your doctor must be careful to consider the effects of that medication on your overnight blood pressure.

Can neuropathy cause unusual sweating?

Yes. Sweating is one way your body regulates your temperature. The sudomotor nerves control where and how much you sweat. If these nerves are damaged, sweating may be absent on your hands and feet and increased on your face and trunk. You may be unaware of the dire condition of your feet and be concerned only with the unusual increase of sweating in your upper body. The most acceptable explanation for this situation is that the body needs to get rid of heat by increasing blood flow and sweating in the upper body to compensate for the loss of peripheral autonomic nerves in the lower body.

In addition, sweating may occur when you are eating, particularly spicy foods, cheese, chocolate, red sausages, red wines, and some soft drinks. (Even people with a normal functioning autonomic nervous system may have head and face sweating when eating spicy food.)

When your sweating response is damaged, your body can't adjust the temperature. This increases your risk for heat stroke. The skin on your feet and hands can get too dry and, as part of the damage process, may not be getting the essential nutrients usually delivered by the blood vessels. Your feet may feel cold. The skin may thicken in response to decreased sweating and lubrication. The thickened skin can crack open and provide a site for bacteria and infections to start. More important is the fact that many of the new devices developed to recognize hypoglycemia rely on sweating as a symptom. These may prove useless if you have autonomic neuropathy—a little-recognized fact.

How is sudomotor nerve damage diagnosed?

Obviously, the symptoms lead to the diagnosis. Your provider can dust you with a special starch powder that turns purple when it gets wet or check your ability to feel warmth in your feet and hands.

What is the treatment for sudomotor neuropathy?

The important thing is to keep your feet and hands healthy and to use lubricating creams and oils after you bathe to keep in the moisture. You should also avoid intense heat and humidity because your body cannot regulate extreme temperatures well. Medications (propantheline hydrobromide, scopolamine patches) may help relieve unusual sweating if it is severe. Your provider may also prescribe a cholinergic blocker to decrease upper-body sweating.

Does autonomic neuropathy affect your body's response to hypoglycemia?

Yes. Autonomic nerves orchestrate your body's symptoms of and response to hypoglycemia. When there is severe autonomic damage, both the capacity to respond to hypoglycemia and the ability to counterregulate it are seriously limited. This can be life-threatening. To counterregulate low blood glucose, your body should release glucagon, epinephrine, growth hormone, cortisol, and glucose from the liver (chapter 2). If it does not, you are not likely to have symptoms of low blood glucose, or *hypoglycemia unawareness*. The autonomic symptoms of hypoglycemia usually are heart palpitations, irregular heartbeat, anxiety, and tingling around the mouth. When you have autonomic neuropathy, your symptoms—when you have any—are more likely due to the shortage of blood glucose in the brain: irritability, tiredness, confusion, forgetfulness, and loss of consciousness.

Furthermore, the epinephrine response is important to counteract hypoglycemia. When you have autonomic neuropathy and repeated episodes of hypoglycemia, this no longer happens. Because of the results of the DCCT, more people practice intensive blood glucose control, and there has been a threefold increase in hypoglycemic episodes requiring the assistance of another person. Although autonomic neuropathy may be delayed by tight control, it puts you more at risk for hypoglycemia, and you may be unaware of it happening. If the hypoglycemia becomes life-threatening, it may be necessary for you to relax your blood glucose goals. Sometimes this will restore your body's responses.

You should also be aware that the symptoms of hypoglycemia will fade over time. The longer you have had diabetes, the more likely you will have at least some degree of hypoglycemia unawareness. To catch hypoglycemia before it goes too low, check your blood glucose level often, especially before you drive.

What should you do if you have hypoglycemia unawareness?

Check blood glucose often and try to determine what your symptoms of hypoglycemia are. If you use insulin, a sulfonylurea, or Prandin, you and your family members and friends should know the symptoms, causes, and treatments of hypoglycemia. You need to have a source of carbohydrate with you always and an up-to-date glucagon kit handy. The kit can be prescribed by your provider, and your family and friends need to be taught how to use it. To prevent hypoglycemia from surprising you, check your blood glucose levels often. You may also want to wear identification jewelry stating that you have diabetes in case hypoglycemia happens when you are away from home or work.

In general, if you have bonafide hypoglycemia unawareness, to avoid life-threatening hypoglycemic episodes, your targets will probably be higher than normal glucose and A1C levels. Often, an insulin pump will help you avoid hypoglycemia. Rapid-acting insulin may help also.

What are focal neuropathies?

Focal neuropathy is damage to a single nerve (*mononeuropathy*), to nerve clusters (*mononeuropathy multiplex*), to nerves in the chest or abdomen (*plexopathy*), or to nerve roots (*radiculopathy*), which often mimics the pain of heart attack or appendicitis. Mononeuropathy affecting nerves to the head is called *cranial neuropathy* and can cause, for example, severe headache, drooping of one side of the face, or double vision. Mononeuropathies in areas where nerves can be trapped or compressed, such as in the wrist and palm, upper arm, elbow, and thigh, are called *entrapment neuropathies*. Carpal tunnel syndrome is an example of an entrapment neuropathy and is fairly common in people with diabetes.

What are mononeuropathies?

Mononeuropathies are lesions in a single nerve that spontaneously heal. Common mononeuropathies involve cranial, thoracic (in the chest), and peripheral nerves. Their onset is sudden and associated with pain, and they generally go away over 6–8 weeks. They must be distinguished from entrapment syndromes, which start slowly, progress, and do not go away without intervention, because the treatment for each is quite different. One example is the condition called *femoral neuropathy*, which involves damage to motor and sensory nerves in the thigh. The symptoms include pain that is sometimes worse at night in the thigh and calf. Muscle weakness can be disabling and can limit hip and knee movements. To distinguish it from sciatica, your provider may have you straighten your leg and raise it. This will be very painful if you have sciatica, but not if you have femoral neuropathy. You should recover completely, but it may last for several years before muscle strength returns to normal.

What is entrapment neuropathy?

The entrapment neuropathies are common in people with diabetes and should be looked for in every patient with symptoms of neuropathy. Common entrapments involve the median nerve in the wrist with impaired sensation in the first three fingers (carpal tunnel syndrome). Ulnar nerve entrapment in the elbow decreases sensation in the little and ring fingers. Damage to the radial nerve (in the upper arm) can cause weakness, loss of sensation on the back of the hand, and dropping of the wrist when extended. Damage to the lateral cutaneous nerve of the thigh causes thigh pain. Damage to the peroneal nerve in the knee causes foot drop. In your foot, medial and lateral plantar nerve entrapments decrease sensation on the inside and outside of the foot, respectively. Finally, tarsal tunnel syndrome may cause numbness and tingling in the foot.

What should you know about carpal tunnel syndrome?

Carpal tunnel syndrome occurs twice as frequently in people with diabetes. This may be related to repeated trauma, metabolic changes, or accumulation of fluid within the confined space of the carpal tunnel. The diagnosis can be confirmed by electrophysiological study, and therapy may be a surgical release. The symptoms may spread to the whole hand and arm in carpal tunnel, and the signs may extend beyond those caused by the trapped nerve. They often involve the thumb, index finger, and one side of the middle finger. The problem is often that the true nature of your trouble goes unrecognized, and an opportunity for successful therapy is missed.

Table 12-2. Self-Care Activities for Diabetic Autonomic Neuropathies

Syndromes	Self-care
Genitourinary Bladder dysfunction	• Empty bladder every 2–3 hours whether you feel the urge or not. • Call your provider at the first sign of a urinary tract infection.
Sexual dysfunction	• Talk with your health care provider about your symptoms.
Gastrointestinal Gastroparesis	• Eat 4–6 small, mostly liquid meals each day. • Eat foods low in fat and fiber. • Take medications before eating, as recommended. • Monitor blood glucose levels often. • Give medications a fair trial.
Intestinal Constipation	• Increase fiber in diet. • Increase fluid intake. • Increase activity. • Use laxatives with caution.
Diarrhea	• Increase fluid intake to prevent dehydration. • Use antidiarrheals with caution.
Cardiovascular dysfunction	• Rise slowly after sitting or lying. After sleeping, sit on the side of the bed and let your feet dangle off the side until you adjust. • Elevate head of bed 30°. • Use elastic stockings as recommended. • Avoid strenuous and aerobic exercise or activity. • Avoid straining or lifting heavy objects. • Stop smoking.
Impaired counterregulation	• Test your blood glucose often, especially before and on breaks during driving on long trips. • Wear diabetes identification. • Teach family, friends, and co-workers how to recognize and treat hypoglycemia. • Keep an up-to-date glucagon kit on hand, and be sure someone around you knows how to use it.
Impaired sweating	• Avoid offending foods. • Use lotion on dry skin. • Use caution when the weather is very hot or humid.
Impaired pupil response	• Turn on the light when entering a dark room. • Use nightlights in dark hallways and bathroom. • Use caution when driving at night.

How is carpal tunnel syndrome treated?

The mainstays of nonsurgical treatment are changing how you use the wrist, special exercises, wearing a wrist splint, and taking anti-inflammatory medications. Surgical treatment consists of sectioning the volar carpal ligament and releasing the entrapped nerve.

What occurs in radiculopathy?

Radiculopathy is damage to a nerve or nerves in the trunk of the body. The primary symptom is pain in the chest (and sometimes the abdomen) that comes on suddenly and is worse at night. The pain does not seem to get worse with exertion as in coughing or exercise. Pain in the chest leads your provider to look first for heart or lung problems. Once these are ruled out, other conditions that can cause similar pain are spinal disk problems, pneumonia, gastrointestinal disease, ulcers, or appendicitis. Ruling out these conditions requires several different diagnostic procedures. Radiculopathy generally goes away within 6 months to 2 years.

Are there self-care activities for living with neuropathy?

Yes. As is repeated throughout this book, maintaining near normal BG levels is most important, but there are other simple things you can do each day to help yourself live better with the effects of neuropathy. See Table 12-2.

Aaron Vinik, MD, PhD, FCP, FACP, contributed to this chapter and the other chapters about neuropathy. Martha M. Funnell, MS, RN, CDE; Douglas A. Greene, MD; Eva L. Feldman, MD, PhD; and Martin J. Stevens, MD also contributed to this chapter.

13

Gastrointestinal Complications

Case study

MK is a 55-year-old woman who has had type 2 diabetes for 10 years. Recently she began to experience heartburn three or four times a week and abdominal bloating and nausea, especially after eating. Her physician prescribed an antibiotic and asked her to avoid foods containing wheat. MK's symptoms did not improve.

Her physician performed a test called *esophagogastroduodenoscopy* (EGD), in which the lining of the esophagus, stomach, and small intestine is examined by looking through a camera in a small flexible tube with a light at the tip. She was given sedatives to help her relax and be comfortable during the test and a local anesthetic spray to numb her throat and prevent gagging. This examination showed moderate inflammation of the esophagus with superficial ulcers called *erosions*. Because she also had bloating and nausea, she underwent a gastric emptying test in which an egg meal was eaten and scans were taken at regular intervals with an external camera. MK's stomach emptying was slower than normal. MK was diagnosed with gastroesophageal reflux disease (GERD) with poor stomach emptying.

She was treated with a medication that reduces the acid in the stomach for the GERD and esophageal inflammation and another medication that speeds up stomach emptying. She showed marked improvement. Regular follow-up visits were useful for adjusting dosage of medication once her symptoms went away.

Case study

MB is a 35-year-old man who has had type 1 diabetes since age 5. He has had neuropathy in his feet and hands and a history of diarrhea of five or six liquid bowel movements a day, alternating with normal bowel movements, for the past year. He consulted his physician because he was unable to control bowel movements and had leakage of stool and soiled underwear when he awoke. Because he did not have any weight loss or other signs of malabsorption, he was treated with diphenoxylate (Lomotil), an antidiarrheal agent.

The diarrhea improved to two or three bowel movements a day, but he still had stool leakage. A rectal examination showed that he had lost some feeling in the rectum. Squeeze pressures in the anal canal were almost normal. Biofeedback training played a role in helping him sense the presence of stool in the rectum and control stool leakage better.

Introduction

Your gastrointestinal (GI) tract is not just a passive biological tube containing digestive juices. It's a very complicated organ, and each section has its own food-processing function. The movement of your GI tract coordinates all these functions. It carries the food that gets delivered at the top through the mixing and digesting processes to the elimination of wastes at the end. This movement is controlled by a sleeve of muscles that surrounds your GI tract. The muscles are controlled by a sophisticated network of nerves. Diabetes can damage these nerves and cause GI problems.

Problems caused by diabetes can occur all along the GI tract, from the mouth to the rectum. The symptoms you experience may give you and your physician some indication of where the problem is occurring. When your stomach is affected, the condition is called *gastroparesis* (stomach paralysis). In people without autonomic neuropathy, liquids empty out of the stomach in about 10–30 minutes and solid foods in 1–2 1/2 hours. With autonomic neuropathy, both liquids and food can remain in the stomach for a longer period. When severe, gastroparesis is one of the most debilitating of all GI complications of diabetes. Other GI tract problems are esophageal disorders, diabetic diarrhea and constipation, and diseases of the pancreas.

What are the symptoms of GI complications?

The symptoms of GI problems caused by diabetes include difficulty swallowing solid or liquid food, heartburn, nausea and vomiting, abdominal pain, constipation, increased need for laxatives, diarrhea, and fecal incontinence (Figure 13-1). Many patients with gastroparesis do not have these symptoms and the only clinical feature is erratic blood glucose control or brittle diabetes.

If your symptoms are difficulty swallowing and heartburn, what condition might you have?

When food gets to your stomach, a sphincter muscle at the bottom of your esophagus closes. This prevents food and acid from coming back up into the esophagus. If muscle contractions are too weak or the sphincter does not close as it should, you will have symptoms of *gastroesophageal reflux*. In gastroesophageal reflux, the contents of the stomach back up into the esophagus. You may experience a feeling that solid or liquid food stops or passes with difficulty through the throat or the chest portion of this tube. You may experience chest pain during or after eating or drinking. You may have heartburn or a burning sensation in your chest or throat after eating a meal, when lying down, or when bending over. These symptoms may awaken

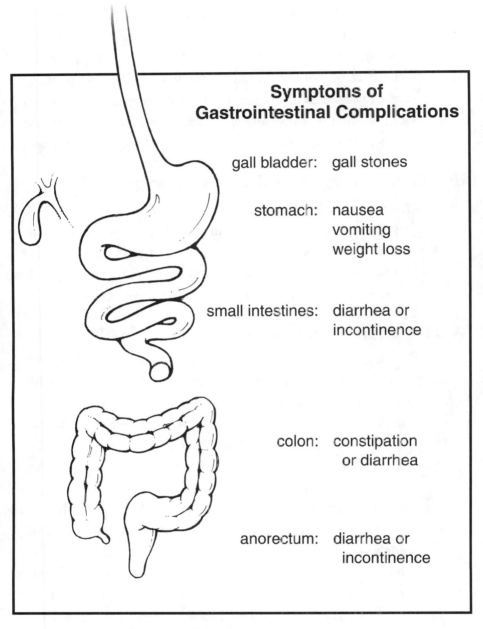

Figure 13-1. Symptoms of gastrointestinal complications.

you from sleep. In some instances, you might only have a bad taste in your mouth and/or throat. Interestingly, two studies have shown that people with type 1 diabetes have a lower incidence of heartburn than people with type 2 and people without diabetes. This may be due to a decrease in stomach acid production in people with type 1 diabetes, whose nerve supply to the stomach acid-producing cells may be damaged.

How does your physician diagnose esophageal reflux?

An upper-GI X ray or examination with a scope can rule out esophagitis (inflammation of the esophagus) or other diseases of the mucous membranes, such as yeast infection or cancer. Chest pain means that you need to have appropriate tests done to rule out poor circulation to the heart as the cause.

What is the treatment for gastroesophageal reflux?

There are nondrug measures that can prevent reflux (heartburn), including lifestyle changes—stopping smoking, losing weight, and avoiding foods that bring on acid reflux, such as caffeine, chocolate, tomato sauce, and high-fat foods. In addition, you should not lie down for 2 hours after a meal, or you should raise your head a few inches more when you do lie down to help prevent acid reflux.

Which drugs to use for the condition depends on the severity and frequency of your symptoms and whether you have esophageal inflammation. Your options range from over-the-counter antacids to H_2 blockers, which decrease stomach acid production, to proton pump inhibitors. Proton pump inhibitors are the strongest gastric acid blockers, and they are more effective at healing esophageal ulcers caused by gastric acid. If you only have occasional symptoms of heartburn, antacids and the lifestyle changes are usually sufficient. When you have heartburn more than once a week, either an H_2 blocker, on a twice-daily regimen, or a proton pump inhibitor is the treatment of choice.

If your symptoms are nausea and vomiting, what condition might you have?

Nausea and vomiting, often accompanied by weight loss, are common symptoms of gastroparesis. These symptoms may be accompanied by abdominal bloating and a feeling of fullness after eating a meal.

Normally, your stomach's slow, steady muscular contractions break food into tiny particles. Then, your stomach pushes these liquids and solids into the small intestine. If you have gastroparesis, the grinding process of the stomach is lost. Foods are not broken up into small pieces, and they remain in the stomach too long. Episodes of nausea and vomiting may last for days or, rarely, months, or they occur in cycles. Blood glucose is probably difficult to control. You may have hypoglycemia whenever the food is not delivered to the small intestine in time to match the insulin you took before the meal.

Gastroparesis typically occurs when you also have other complications of diabetes such as retinopathy, nephropathy, and peripheral neuropathy. Other symptoms of autonomic damage are sluggish pupil responses, lack of sweating, facial sweating while eating certain foods, dizziness on standing, impotence, diminished ejaculation, and poor function of the bladder with recurring infections.

How does your physician diagnose gastroparesis?

Your physician must rule out conditions causing symptoms similar to those of delayed stomach emptying, such as chronic peptic ulcer disease, cancer, or uremia, and side effects of medications. Some of the medications that delay stomach emptying are those that are used to treat high blood pressure and depression.

To make a definite diagnosis of gastroparesis, a stomach-emptying test using solid food should be performed. During this test, your blood glucose must not be greater than 240 mg/dl because hyperglycemia by itself slows gastric emptying and the results of the test would simply reflect your high blood glucose. After you eat a radioactive meal, the level of radioactivity in your stomach is measured at different times to measure the ability of your stomach to empty food. You might also have a gastroscopy, where the doctor looks into your stomach using a scope that carries a tiny camera.

About one-third of patients with type 1 diabetes have some form of eating disorder. When this becomes significant to the extent of anorexia or bulimia (see chapter 16), then gastroparesis can develop and create a vicious cycle.

In the first 3–5 years with type 2 diabetes, you may be bothered by rapid liquid-phase gastric emptying, a condition that may slow the emptying of more solid foods from the stomach and contribute to diarrhea.

What is the treatment for gastroparesis?

Treatment for delayed stomach emptying includes changing your diet to eat small meals more often and avoiding high-fat foods and uncooked vegetables. You may try a drug that stimulates your stomach to contract and empty itself. If you have severe nausea and vomiting that lead to dehydration, you are in danger of diabetic ketoacidosis (see chapter 1) and should be hospitalized. You may need to have your stomach pumped to remove the contents quickly. Intravenous fluids should be given to correct metabolic imbalances such as ketoacidosis, uremia, hypoglycemia/hyperglycemia, or low blood potassium levels. Parenteral nutrition (a feeding tube bypassing the stomach) may be necessary if you are malnourished.

If one drug doesn't work for you, your doctor may try a different one or a combination of drugs. Sometimes a drug may be effective for weeks or months only to apparently wear off. Or the side effects may bother you too much. Your doctor may raise the dosage or try a new drug. Some people have gastroparesis for years, and then it seems to go away. Others have milder symptoms off and on all of their lives. If you have symptoms, don't give up. You may need to be referred to a specialist.

To get control of your blood glucose levels, you may need to check your blood glucose more often and when they're high, bring them down with insulin. Eating small meals throughout the day rather than a few large meals often helps. Avoid a high-fat, high-fiber diet. Avoid foods containing difficult-to-digest material, such as legumes, lentils, and citrus fruits. Undigested food may form "tumors" known as bezoars. These bezoars will worsen your symptoms of fullness, nausea, and abdominal discomfort, and they can be very difficult for a doctor to remove.

If you have heartburn, will you need an EGD?

It is not necessary for every case of heartburn to be diagnosed with an EGD. Your physician will probably treat your symptoms first. You only have an EGD in cases where the diagnosis is not clear or the first treatments have not brought any improvement.

If your symptom is diarrhea, what might the condition be?

Diarrhea is a particularly difficult problem in about 5% of people with diabetes. It can be severe and usually occurs in patients with a long history of diabetes and insulin use. Diarrhea can occur at any time and with little warning, but it commonly occurs at night. It may be associated with fecal incontinence, which is leakage of stool without the feeling of urgency to have a bowel movement.

The cause of diabetic diarrhea is not well understood. It is probably related to diabetic nerve damage (autonomic neuropathy). Neuropathy can affect the muscles that move food through the bowel and absorb fluid from the digested food. Neuropathy may also damage the anal sphincter muscles and interfere with normal sensation in the rectum. That's why people don't feel the need to have a bowel movement.

Of course, it may be caused by dietetic foods containing sorbitol (an artificial sweetener). It might be associated with conditions that disrupt absorption of nutrients, such as too much bacteria in the small intestine, celiac sprue (an unusual reaction to wheat), or more rarely, a problem with bile acid, which helps you digest fats. Very rarely, it is associated with low production of pancreatic enzymes. Certainly, this symptom is distressing enough to keep many people at home and very concerned, so the sooner treatment begins, the better.

How is diabetic diarrhea diagnosed?

If neuropathy is the cause of the diarrhea, sensation is reduced around the anus, and this can be detected with a pin. Rectal examination shows a lax sphincter that does not contract around an inserted finger. There is loss of the anal wink reflex, which is contraction of the anus in a "wink" when the skin around the anus is stroked. And there is loss of the bulbocavernosus reflex, in which the anus can be seen or felt to contract when the glans penis is squeezed between the fingers.

Before any tests are performed, you and your physician should check your diet for foods containing sorbitol (such as some sugar-free candies), excess caffeine, laxatives, and magnesium-based antacids, which are probably the most common causes of diarrhea in people with diabetes. Also, medications such as metformin can cause diarrhea.

What is the treatment for diabetic diarrhea?

Your physician may have you try a wheat gluten–free diet to see if that improves the condition or check you for food allergies. You may take a broad-spectrum antibiotic to deal with overgrowth of bacteria in the bowel. If you have small intestine bacterial overgrowth (more than 100,000 organisms per milliliter), you will be put on an antibiotic for 10 days. If that doesn't help, you may be given an antidiarrheal drug such as diphenoxylate (Lomotil).

If your condition does not improve, your physician can rule out bacteria growing in your small intestine or celiac sprue with an upper-GI endoscopy to gather fluid for small intestinal bacterial cultures and to look at and biopsy the small bowel lining. You may or may not need to do a 72-hour stool collection to test the fat content to check pancreatic enzyme action. You would be given pancreatic enzymes for pancreatic insufficiency in the rare event that this was the cause of your problem. In case of bile acid malabsorption (also very rare), cholestyramine, which binds bile acids, or loperamide (Imodium), which slows the transit time in the small intestine, may control diarrhea.

To treat fecal incontinence, first work on the diarrhea. It often disappears when the diarrhea improves. Many patients do not tell their physicians about the fecal incontinence, or they just call it diarrhea. It is crucial for patients and physicians to distinguish between the two conditions because specialized treatment for incontinence can help greatly.

Successful treatment for fecal incontinence includes biofeedback techniques and sphincter muscle training (also called Kegel exercises). A nurse educator or physical therapist can teach you how to squeeze and relax your sphincter muscles. It involves squeezing as though you're trying to prevent urine or stool from coming out. Get in the habit of doing this simple exercise several times a day, say, when you're at a stop light or during TV commercials. In people with good rectal sensation, sphincter-strengthening exercises and biofeedback techniques are successful 70% of the time. The drug octreotide acetate (Sandostatin), which is injected under the skin immediately before meals, is sometimes necessary and works well.

What is constipation?

Constipation is defined as a decrease in frequency of bowel movements to less than three per week, presence of hard stool, or need for straining. Patients with constipation may also need to assume a contorted posture such as bending down to eliminate the stool, have a sense of incomplete evacuation, have rectal discomfort, or frequently need laxatives or enemas. Constipation is probably the most common GI complication of diabetes. It affects 25% of people with diabetes and more than 50% of those with neuropathy.

Typically, constipation comes and goes and may alternate with episodes of diarrhea. Constipation is most commonly caused either by slow colonic transit—that is, the fecal material takes too long to pass through the colon—or by some obstruction at the rectum. Obstruction can be caused by anal sphincters and/or pelvic muscles not working correctly. Pelvic muscles play an important role in normal bowel movements. If they are uncoordinated or weak, they can cause constipation. Not drinking enough water or eating enough food with fiber and not getting enough exercise can cause you to be constipated. Medications and other illnesses can also cause constipation.

What is the treatment for constipation?

Simple measures will improve constipation. Drink plenty of water during the day. Get regular exercise, which will help intestinal movement. Your bowels tend to move after a meal; take advantage of this gastrocolonic reflex by sitting on the toilet 30 minutes or so after a meal.

You should eat 20–35 grams of fiber per day, unless you have gastroparesis. Fiber is found in fruits, vegetables, legumes (beans, peas, and lentils), and whole grains. Oats, beans, peas, fresh fruits, and brown rice are great choices and should be eaten in amounts consistent with your meal plan.

Food is your best source of fiber. Medications such as stool softeners or psyllium are available over the counter and may be effective when combined with other self-care measures. Excess fiber can aggravate constipation and cause gas, so you should increase the fiber in your diet gradually. Laxatives and antidiarrheal agents should be used with caution. Your body may start to depend on laxatives, and overuse of antidiarrheals can cause constipation.

If increasing dietary fiber does not relieve the constipation, a proctosigmoidoscopy enables your physician to examine the rectum and intestines with a flexible tube with a light at the end. It is less likely, but you may have a barium enema (an X ray of your intestines taken after you've been given an enema containing a soft metal called barium) or colonoscopy to evaluate your condition. A colonoscopy enables the physician to examine the lining of your colon.

If the mucous membrane of your rectum and colon is normal, the physician may evaluate your muscles for the ability to expel stool using a simple rectal examination such as the one described above. Other tests are anorectal manometry, and evaluation of the pelvic floor muscles or the nerves supplying the muscles of the anus and rectum. If pelvic nerve and muscle function are normal, then an X ray or gamma camera test that measures the speed of movement of solid matter through the colon may be done.

If pelvic function is normal, include fiber or laxatives such as milk of magnesia in your diet. If these measures fail to help, you may need an enema program. In patients with slow colonic transit, medications that increase colonic motility such as bisacodyl (Dulcolax), promotility agents such as cisapride (see Table 13-1), or glycerin suppositories may be helpful.

What does the symptom of chronic abdominal pain mean?

People with diabetes obviously have the same causes of abdominal pain as the general population. However, you have

Table 13-1. Prokinetic Medicines

Drug	Action	Comments
Metoclopramide (Reglan)	Decreases a gastric inhibitor (dopamine pathway) allowing the autonomic nerves to work uninhibited	Has separate effects on the brain to decrease nausea
Bethanechol (Urecholine)	Directly stimulates the autonomic nervous system pathway	May cause sweating and be confused with hypoglycemia if too large a dose is given
Erythromycin	Directly acts on muscles of GI tract like a gut hormone called motilin	An antibiotic—often loses its potency as a GI stimulator in a few months
Domperidone	Works like metoclopramide	No effects on the brain
Cisapride (Propulsid)	Directly stimulates smooth muscles in gut and stimulates local nervous system pathway	Can't use with erythromycin
Sandostatin	Decreases a gastric inhibitor (GIP, a gut hormone)	Needs to be given subcutaneously (under the skin)

an increased risk of developing gallstone disease. It is probably because the gallbladder, which stores bile from the liver, does not contract as much, so bile pools in it, forms sludge, and, finally, makes stones. The pain is caused when the gallbladder attempts to push bile out and the stones get caught in the opening or too many stones are formed. Gallbladder pain may worsen after a meal or in the middle of the night and may be accompanied by nausea or vomiting.

Pain may also be caused by impaired circulation to the intestines resulting from atherosclerosis of those blood vessels. If the nerves supplying the chest and abdominal wall are affected by diabetic neuropathy, you may feel pain in the girdle area due to diabetic radiculopathy (see chapter 12). Other causes are referral pain from the heart and gastroparesis.

In conclusion

Although there are several treatments for GI complications of diabetes, management has been only partially successful. Maintain normal glucose control and control symptoms because there are no treatments to reverse the neuropathy that plays a role in causing these GI abnormalities.

Michael Camilleri, MD; Dordaneh Maleki, MD; and Jeffrey L. Barnett, MD, contributed to this chapter.

14

Infection and Diabetes

Introduction

Infectious diseases can be caused by a large variety of microorganisms, including viruses, bacteria, fungi, and parasites. People with diabetes will get the same infections as everyone else, but certain infections tend to occur more frequently or are more severe in people with diabetes. This chapter explains how and why infections may present a special problem for you.

How does your immune system deal with infections?

Our bodies are surrounded by and colonized with vast numbers of microorganisms that would like to use us as a source of food and housing. To prevent ourselves from being infected, we have developed a remarkably effective system of defenses. Infections develop only when these defenses are breached. The first lines of defense are anatomical and physiological barriers, such as our skin and the acid in our stomach. In addition, we have a complex inner immune system that helps recognize invading microorganisms and destroy them.

White blood cells are produced in your bone marrow and circulate in the bloodstream until they are needed to fight an invading microorganism. These cells are attracted to an infected area by chemicals that are released when tissue damage occurs.

What are the symptoms of infection?

When an organism such as a bacteria or virus enters your body, it triggers a series of events designed to fight the invasion. This process produces many of the classic signs and symptoms of inflammation, such as pain, tenderness, redness, warmth, and swelling. Pain is caused by chemicals produced by the body to attract white blood cells, by the release of toxins from the invading germ, and by the destruction of the tissue under attack. These chemicals and toxins are also responsible for the heat associated with an infection. As more chemicals are released, the small blood vessel (capillary) beds near the infection dilate (expand) to allow more white blood cells to enter the infected area. This increase in blood supply causes the warmth and redness that is associated with an infection.

As the infection progresses, a thick, cloudy fluid called *pus* may form. This is made up of white blood cells, germs, tissue debris, and fluid from the blood vessels. Unlike the clear yellow drainage in many uninfected wounds, the presence of pus should be taken as evidence of an infection. As pus accumulates, it may cause a swelling called an *abscess.*

How are infections and blood glucose control connected?

Poor blood glucose control over long periods appears to increase your risk for developing certain infections. In addition, blood glucose can rise dramatically when the body is under stress, such as when it is fighting an infection. Among the responses to stress are increases in the secretion of various hormones, including cortisol and glucagon (see chapters 1 and 2). These, in turn, increase the release of glucose from the liver, so the blood glucose level goes even higher.

Does insulin help you deal with infections?

Insulin helps lower blood glucose. When patients who use insulin are admitted to the hospital for treatment of a severe illness, they may require increased insulin doses to manage their blood glucose levels. High blood glucose levels impair the white cells' ability to digest and kill bacteria. Patients with type 2 diabetes who do not use insulin may temporarily need insulin to reduce their hyperglycemia, but once the infection or stress is under control, insulin therapy is usually no longer required.

Are people with diabetes more likely to have immune problems?

At least three factors are important. First, your immune system's production and use of many key infection-fighting components, such as white blood cells and antibodies, is impaired. Second, there are complications of diabetes, including both large and small blood vessel disease, that hinder your body's ability to deliver these infection fighters. The third factor resides in your ability to sense the infection. Nerve damage may make you unable to sense changes associated with an ongoing infection. By the time you notice the signs and symptoms of inflammation, the infection can be quite severe.

Can normal microorganisms cause infections in people with diabetes?

Bacteria and fungi that are routinely found on certain parts of your body are called *normal flora*. Areas where these organisms grow in colonies include the skin, mouth, and intestinal tract. These organisms actually help prevent infection. but the normal flora, like other microorganisms, can also cause infections. This may occur when there are too many by overgrowth at a site where they are normally found (for example, oral thrush caused by overgrowth of a common yeastlike fungus called *Candida*) or by invading a site where they are not normally found (for example, skin bacteria infecting bone at the base of an open foot ulcer). Infections, unlike normal colony growth, are characterized by the presence of pus or by the signs of inflammation. Diabetes appears to put you more at risk for infections with organisms that rarely cause infections in people who do not have diabetes.

How are the different types of infection diagnosed?

Many different microorganisms can cause infection, but bacteria are the most important. Only about a dozen are relatively common. We classify bacteria by several characteristics. Two of the most useful are *1*) whether the bacteria need oxygen (aerobic) or do not need oxygen (anaerobic) to grow and *2*) whether they appear purple (gram-positive) or pink (gram-negative) on slides containing specially stained smears of body specimens. These classifications help predict the course the infection is likely to take and the most appropriate antibiotics to use for treatment. The specific organism causing an infection is identified by culturing (growing in the lab) a specimen from the affected area—for example, urine, pus, or mucus. The most frequent bacterial types causing infections in patients with diabetes are aerobic gram-positive organisms, specifically a bacteria type of germ called *Staphylococcus*. Aerobic gram-negative organisms are the most common in urinary tract infections. Anaerobic organisms (both gram-positive and gram-negative) are usually found with other bacteria in deep soft-tissue infections. They are often associated with a foul odor. Each antibiotic acts against a specific group of organisms. Organisms that grow on the cultures can be tested against various antibiotics to determine how susceptible they are to each one.

Are any infections more common in people with diabetes?

People with diabetes are more likely to develop several specific types of infections. Foot ulcers are common and dangerous (chapter 3). Those infections that are most common or best studied are urinary tract infections, lower-leg infections, foot ulcers, malignant external otitis (an external ear infection), rhinocerebral mucormycosis (a fungal sinus infection), and fungal nail infections. For skin infections, see chapter 15.

What type of urinary tract infections might you be more likely to develop?

You are more likely to develop infections in the urinary tract called *bacteriuria*, *cystitis*, or *pyelonephritis*.

Bacteriuria

Urine is normally sterile (free from or contains only a small number of bacteria). Infections of the urinary tract (bladder and kidney) are, however, probably the most common type of infection in people with diabetes. The term *bacteriuria* means a high number—100,000 per milliliter or greater—of bacteria present in the urine, as detected by a culture. This condition is more common in people with diabetes, especially women. Factors that further increase your chance of developing bacteriuria include being elderly, having abnormalities of genital or urinary structures (such as an enlarged prostate gland), or having diabetes longer than 10–15 years.

Bacteriuria may not cause symptoms, discomfort, or disease. Its importance is that it makes you more likely to develop an infection of the bladder (*cystitis*) or the kidneys (*pyelonephritis*). It usually does not require antibiotic therapy, except in people who have a bladder dysfunction or an obstruction of urinary flow or those who are pregnant, have immune system problems, or are scheduled to undergo an invasive procedure on the urinary tract, such as bladder catheterization. The benefit to anyone else taking antibiotics for this condition is outweighed by the potential side effects of taking the antibiotic and growing antibiotic-resistant bacteria.

For people who have repeated urinary tract infections with symptoms, long-term daily doses of antibiotics help prevent bacteriuria, but reinfection occurs quickly when you stop taking the medicine. Many different antibiotics can be used for therapy and prevention. The choice depends on the organisms that are likely to be causing the infection, the site of the infection, the frequency of the side effects, the cost of the drugs, the patient's preferences, and other factors.

Cystitis

When bacteriuria causes symptoms of bladder inflammation, you have cystitis. Symptoms of acute (sudden-onset) cystitis include pain or burning on urination, increased frequency of urination, pain over the bladder (above the pubic area), and sometimes fever. Your urine may be cloudy, have a foul odor, or even contain some blood. Most bladder infections are caused by bacteria and respond within a few days to oral antibiotics. Antibiotics are usually given for 3–10 days. Patients with diabetes are also more likely to have urinary tract infections caused by fungi, which require special, anti-fungal agents. Fungi can occasionally form a large mass called a *fungus ball*. These can occur anywhere in the urinary tract and may require surgical removal. Rarely, patients develop a severe form of bladder infection that is characterized by air in the bladder wall and is called *emphysematous cystitis*. This usually requires hospitalization and possibly surgery.

Pyelonephritis

Infected urine from the bladder can go up the ureters (the tubes connecting the bladder to the kidneys) to cause an infection of the kidneys called pyelonephritis. Acute pyelonephritis is typically characterized by fever. chills, nausea, vomiting, and severe side or upper-back pain. These symptoms may occur at the same time as, or soon after, symptoms of cystitis.

Patients with pyelonephritis may be treated on an outpatient basis if they are not experiencing severe symptoms such as high fever, severe high blood glucose levels, or vomiting. If they do have these symptoms, hospitalization with intravenous therapy is needed for a few days. The total duration of antibiotic therapy is usually 2 weeks.

If your health care provider suspects that you have pyelonephritis, especially if your symptoms have persisted for several days, an abdominal X ray should be done to look for *emphysematous pyelonephritis*. This unusual but serious complication is diagnosed by the presence of gas in the kidneys. It is estimated that 70–90% of all cases of emphysematous pyelonephritis occur in patients with diabetes, perhaps because the bacteria or fungi that cause it use the abundant sugar present in their tissues to produce the gas. As with emphysematous cystitis, this infection requires immediate hospitalization. Other complications of kidney infections include infection of the tissues surrounding the kidney and death of tissue in the kidneys. After an episode of pyelonephritis has been treated, most patients should be evaluated for abnormalities of the urinary tract that may make them more likely to get infections in the future. This evaluation may include an ultrasound examination of the kidneys, measurement of urinary flow, an excretory urogram (an X ray with an injection of dye), or cystoscopy (looking into the bladder with a special instrument).

What is malignant external otitis?

Malignant, or invasive, *external otitis* is a serious type of external ear infection that occurs almost exclusively in patients with diabetes. The name refers to the severity of infection; it is not a cancer. This infection begins in the external ear canal, then involves the soft tissue adjacent to the ear, and may eventually spread to the bone located near the ear canal. Patients with diabetes who develop this type of bacterial infection are typically older (more than 65 years old), are predominately male, and have long-standing diabetes.

Signs of malignant external otitis include severe, persistent earache, festering and sometimes foul smelling ear discharge, and possibly hearing loss. As the infection progresses, it may involve the base of the skull or even the facial nerve, which may cause drooping of facial muscles. Patients may also have systemic signs of infection, such as fever, and elevated glucose levels and white blood cell count. Diagnosis may be aided by special X rays or scans.

Once diagnosed, therapy includes long-term (more than 6 weeks) antibiotics. Surgical debridement of infected tissue or bone may also be necessary. Despite appropriate therapy, the infection may come back.

What is rhinocerebral mucormycosis?

This is an uncommon fungal infection that occurs in people with diabetes, especially those who have had episodes of ketoacidosis (chapter 1). It involves your nasal sinuses or the palate of your mouth. The fungi that cause this infection can grow rapidly in the presence of high glucose and in an acid environment—such as ketoacidosis. This infection can be life-threatening and advances rapidly.

The first symptoms are usually pain in your eyes or face, followed by yellowish white or blood-tinged nasal discharge, swelling around the eyes, increased tearing, visual blurring, and sinus or nasal tenderness. Physical examination may disclose a darkening or ulceration in the nasal passages or palate, and X-ray examinations help confirm the diagnosis.

Therapy must be started early and be aggressive to prevent spread of the infection to the brain. You need surgical removal of the dead and infected tissue and antifungal and antibiotic medicines.

What is onychomycosis?

Onychomycosis is a fungal infection of the nails, most commonly of the great toenail. It can spread to the other nails of the feet and hands. The fungus causes the nails to become rough, thickened, and yellow. Eventually, the entire nail may become soft and crumbly and may fall off. What disturbs people most is the appearance of the nail, but the infection can lead to ulcers and infection of the toe itself.

Nail fungus can be treated by oral antifungal drugs. See your physician for a fungal culture and possible treatment with prescription oral drugs such as terbinafine (Lamisil) or itraconazole (Sporanox). Your physician must take a culture from the nail and the skin beneath the nail before giving you any of the newer oral antifungal agents. Several of these drugs have side effects that you should discuss with your provider. These new drugs are used for 12 weeks of therapy with a success rate of up to 80% of nails treated. However, the fungal infection frequently returns. Also, it takes a new toenail 18 to 24 months to grow out normally after the fungus has been treated.

How can you avoid infections and disease?

The most important way to prevent infections from developing is to keep your blood glucose levels as near normal as possible. The next most important measure is part of the first—eat well-balanced meals. When you don't eat enough vegetables and whole grains and you eat too much white flour and sugary foods, your body environment is acidic, which encourages microorganisms to grow.

Are there vaccines that can help you prevent infections?

Some vaccines can protect you against infections caused by viruses. As you get older, you should protect yourself from the flu virus by getting the new flu vaccine each year, unless you are allergic to eggs. Yearly vaccinations are necessary because the viruses that cause the flu change frequently. If you are 65 years or older, you should get a one-time shot that protects against 23 of the most common strains of pneumonia. In some cases, it might be necessary to get another vaccination; check with your physician to see if yours needs to be updated. Flu vaccine is about 70% effective, and the pneumonia vaccine is about 60% effective, but both are very good at reducing the risk of serious infection, complications, and death. It is also becoming more common for people to be vaccinated against hepatitis B, a disease that can damage your liver and is becoming more widespread. Babies are now routinely given this vaccine in the first days after birth.

If you travel to other countries, you can contact your local travel agent, public health department, or the Centers for Disease Control to learn which vaccinations are recommended for your protection in the countries you'll be visiting. Again, the hepatitis B vaccine is recommended, as is a tetanus shot if you haven't had one in the past 10 years. Infections can worsen more rapidly in tropical conditions, so be extra watchful for the signs and symptoms of infection, and seek medical care early.

Benjamin A. Lipsky, MD, and Paul D. Baker contributed to this chapter.

15

Diabetes and Skin

Introduction

It is difficult to say whether diabetes is the cause of many skin conditions, but there are certain conditions that are more common in people with diabetes. By and large, they are not serious. Still, it is important to check your skin often for color changes or damage.

Are you more likely to have waxy, thick skin?

People with diabetes commonly have thickening of the skin. It may relate to accelerated aging or fraying of the elastic tissue. Under the microscope, diabetic thick skin shows increased thickness, disorganization of collagen bundles (the connective tissue of the skin), and deposits of sugarlike substances. Thickening of the skin and stiffness in the tendons in your hands may decrease the joint mobility and limit how far you can extend your fingers, but it is painless. This is more common when blood glucose control is poor. You can check for this condition by trying to put your hand flat on a tabletop or by putting your hands together in a praying position. If you cannot straighten your fingers out completely, you may have this condition. The skin often has a yellow, waxy appearance and loses some of its surface flexibility. Improving blood glucose control has been shown to help with this condition and make the skin less thick. Otherwise, there is no known treatment.

People with diabetes are also more at risk for developing a joint mobility problem called *frozen shoulder* (*adhesive capsulitis*). If you have difficulty or pain raising your arm or using your shoulder, see your health care provider, because the condition is easier to treat at the beginning with physical therapy. Once the shoulder is completely "frozen," the condition must run its course, which can take a year or more.

What is Dupuytren's contracture?

When the tendons attached to the fingers become contracted, the fingers gradually become permanently bent, and you are unable to extend them. This is referred to as *Dupuytren's contracture*. It requires surgical correction.

Is yellow skin associated with diabetes?

It has been suggested that people with diabetes may have a yellowish tint to their skin because a product of the metabolism of glucose has a yellow hue. Your fingernails and toenails may also become yellow. The cause, again, is not known but may be a byproduct of glucose metabolism. Some people with diabetes, especially elderly people, develop yellow nails because of peripheral vascular disease or fungus. However, about half of the cases of yellow nails in people with diabetes have no known cause. The first sign may be a brown or yellow color on the nail. Later, all the nails can turn bright yellow. It is generally harmless and does not require treatment.

What is diabetic dermopathy?

Diabetic dermopathy refers to small, round, colored spots on the lower leg, usually found on the shins. They are more common in older men with diabetes and, in some studies, have been documented in 70% of men with diabetes over

60 years of age. They are the most common skin sign of diabetes but, on occasion, may be observed in people who do not have diabetes.

Diabetic dermopathy starts as small pink spots that gradually turn brown. They are approximately the size of an eraser on the end of a pencil, and the skin may be thinned with tiny scales on top. Although the cause is unknown, trauma, especially in people with neuropathy, may lead to this condition. It is believed that the effect of high glucose levels on collagen in the skin is responsible for the brown color. The spots will disappear spontaneously; however, new individual or clusters of spots often appear nearby. No treatment is necessary.

What is necrobiosis lipoidica diabeticorum (NLD)?

Necrobiosis lipoidica diabeticorum is the name of the red-yellow spots that may appear on the lower legs of people with diabetes—usually those with type 1 diabetes. *Necrobiosis* means the breakdown of collagen in the skin, which can be observed under the microscope in samples of tissue (biopsies) from these spots. *Lipoidica* refers to the yellow color, similar to that of fat, that is seen in the center of these spots when the surface skin has thinned. *Diabeticorum* indicates that diabetes is commonly associated with the appearance of this condition. Sometimes, this skin condition may appear before there are any clinical signs or symptoms of diabetes. The condition favors young adults and occurs more often in women than in men.

This condition is not common; it occurs in only 3 of every 1,000 people with diabetes each year. NLD starts with red bumps that gradually join together and enlarge. Those spots then develop a thin yellow center, the skin becomes shiny and transparent, and you can see tiny blood vessels under the surface. The most common location of NLD is the shin (in 90% of patients), but lesions can occur on the scalp, face, arms, and body. In one in three people, the area will become an open sore or ulcer, especially if it is on the lower leg. The ulcer results from the very thin and fragile skin over the sore. Such an ulcer should be monitored by your health care provider.

The cause of this condition is unknown. Changes in small blood vessels, an immune system response, or an injury to the skin may all play contributing roles in this condition. These spots are chronic, but they disappear spontaneously in 10–20% of cases. It is common for them to return.

If you do not have an ulcer, you may only need to protect the area from being bumped by other people or objects (wearing shin pads) and turning on the light before you get up at night to walk around. Your doctor may have you apply a steroid cream and a light bandage. It is not clear whether improved blood glucose control can help. Applying topical steroid cream and covering it with an airtight bandage or injecting steroids into the dermis (second layer of the skin) may help control the formation of new thick red areas in the skin. Once the skin has thinned, use only topical moisturizing creams. Some oral medications have been used in research studies, including low-dose aspirin and the antiplatelet drug dipyridamole. Further studies are necessary to show whether routine use of these drugs is beneficial. Ulcers, of course, require prompt treatment.

Cosmetic treatment is often important to patients, especially young women. A green-based waterproof cosmetic cream may cover areas of discoloration. Seek expert advice from an experienced cosmetologist to do your "leg colors" with a green base and added color.

What is granuloma annulare?

Granuloma annulare is an inflammatory skin disease. It is characterized by ring-shaped sores that form from flesh-colored, red, or red-brown bumps. The skin in the center of these lesions may be normal or red and is flat. The most common form of this condition appears on the hands or feet of children and young adults. There are no other symptoms, and generally, the condition limits itself.

The condition may take other forms. If it spreads across the arms, neck, and trunk, it is called generalized granuloma annulare. We do not know what causes this disease. Treatment is similar to that for NLD and includes topical and injected steroids and niacinamide. This is usually a temporary condition.

What is scleredema?

Scleredema is a rare disorder of thickened skin on the back, shoulders, and neck. (It is different from the serious disorder *scleroderma*, which has a similar-sounding name.) You may not be able to see all the areas involved, but the surface skin may look like the skin of an orange. Less common areas to check for this condition include the face, upper arms, abdomen, lower back, and tongue.

In children who may or may not have diabetes, scleredema is usually preceded by streptococcal or viral infections. A few weeks later, the child may have hardened shiny skin on his or her neck, upper back, or shoulders that cannot be wrinkled or pressed together to make folds. The condition is painless, and any symptoms appear to result from the limitation of movement by the thickened skin. This disease usually heals spontaneously but can take as long as 18 months.

In people with diabetes, scleredema is a bit different. This change is more common in men who are overweight. It may involve more areas of the body. You may have decreased sensation to pain or light touch in these areas. It may be accompanied by redness of the skin that might be misdiagnosed as treatment-resistant cellulitis. This type of scleredema is less likely to go away on its own, and there is no treatment for it.

Can you get a blister without an injury to the skin?

Yes. Although it is uncommon, people with diabetes sometimes do develop blisters without any apparent cause. In a condition called *bullosis diabeticorum*, clear blisters appear spontaneously on your forearms, fingers, feet, or toes. The blisters arise from normal skin, range in size, are painless, and usually go away in 2–4 weeks. They become dark or black as they heal. They are common in people who have loss of nerve sensation (neuropathy) and in middle-aged to elderly patients with long-standing diabetes. Other than local care, there is no specific treatment needed. Don't break the blister. Let it dry up by itself, but notify your physician about it.

What are xanthomas?

Xanthomas are skin bumps that can accompany poorly controlled blood glucose levels and high blood fat levels—high triglycerides and high cholesterol. They most often appear on the elbows, knees, buttocks, or the site of an injury. Eruptive xanthomas can appear suddenly, and the lesions are usually 4–6 mm in diameter and yellow with a red base. The bumps are firm, not tender, and it is rare for them to break or to cause an ulcer. Biopsy (tissue sample) findings indicate collections of lipids (fats) within the second layer of skin.

Improving blood glucose control and lowering blood fat levels makes xanthomas disappear. Sometimes insulin is required to correct the underlying causes.

Xanthelasma palpebrarum is the name of a xanthoma on the eyelid. Xanthelasmas are the most common type of xanthoma. They may be caused by high blood fats (high cholesterol) and are a sign to your provider to check your cholesterol level. They begin as small yellow-orange bumps, grow, thicken, and can eventually cover the entire eyelid. They are more likely to occur in women than in men.

What is acanthosis nigricans?

In *acanthosis nigricans*, velvety tan to dark brown areas are seen on the sides of the neck, sides of the body, armpits, and groin. Additional possible locations include joints of the hand and fingers, elbows, and knees. This condition may be associated with obesity and type 2 diabetes with high insulin resistance. Patients with this condition frequently require high doses of insulin. Weight loss and improved blood glucose control improve the condition. Otherwise, the only treatment is topical agents such as retinoic acid and urea, if you want to improve the cosmetic appearance.

What is vitiligo?

Vitiligo is a condition of patches of skin that have lost pigment and have no color. If you get a suntan, these areas do not tan. There are fungal infections that can look like vitiligo, so see your provider for a proper diagnosis. Commonly, it affects the trunk of the body, but it may also appear at openings such as the nostrils, eyes, and mouth. Vitiligo may be an immune disorder, and there is no treatment except to cover it with makeup. It is more common in people with type 1 diabetes.

Are you more likely to have itchy skin with diabetes?

You will not necessarily have itchy skin. When it affects feet and legs, it may be very bothersome and cause you to scratch a great deal. This is dangerous because scratching can damage the skin. Elderly patients are usually the ones who have this problem, but it can be resolved by using moisturizing or steroid cream. The itching may be due to an irritation of sensory nerve endings. Diabetes can seriously affect your kidneys, and itchy skin may be one of the symptoms of kidney complications (see chapter 9). Uremia, or elevated levels of urea in the blood, can also cause itching. Maintaining close-to-normal blood glucose levels and kidney function may help.

Over time, the condition may go away on its own. Sometimes medicine (such as Periactin) is needed.

People with diabetes are more likely to develop *herpes zoster*, or shingles, a disease involving the nerves that causes very painful itching. Improving nutrition and achieving better blood glucose control can help.

What is a glucagonoma?

A *glucagonoma* is a tumor affecting the pancreas islet cells that produce the hormone glucagon. It can cause a red or brownish red skin rash called *necrolytic migratory erythema*. These skin lesions can appear on the lower abdomen, buttocks, hands, feet, or legs. This condition is chronic and may precede the discovery of the tumor by several years. The tongue may appear smooth and bright red. Patients with this condition also have anemia, diarrhea, and weight loss. Of course, the tumor needs to be removed or treated, which will resolve the rash, but glucose given in saline has been found to treat the rash successfully.

What are some of the common skin infections associated with diabetes?

People with higher levels of glucose in their blood are more likely to have skin infections. Having some of the complications of diabetes, such as blood vessel narrowing, will also contribute to the occurrence of these infections. *Candida* (or yeast) infections, bacterial infections, and other fungal infections of the skin are discussed below.

Candida infections

Candida is a yeast that will infect moist areas of the skin or mucous membranes in areas such as the mouth, vagina, or rectum. *Candida* infections appear differently in various regions of the body. Inside the mouth, white, curdlike growths appear on the tongue or inner surface of the cheeks. When these are scraped, the surface often bleeds. At the corner of the mouth, yeast infections are often red and moist. The skin in body folds under the arms, under the breasts, on the sides of the groin, and around the anus also provide warmth and moisture that attracts *Candida* infections. In these locations a bright red spot is often surrounded by smaller dotted spots that may have central yellow pustules. In the vagina, *Candida* infections are similar to those in the mouth, with a white curdlike appearance that will bleed when removed. Infections in the vagina and other areas of the body are often extremely itchy.

The treatment of yeast infections is aided by good blood glucose control. In the mouth, nystatin solution (an antiyeast antibiotic) may be used in a swish-and-spit technique three or four times a day for 5–7 days. Clotrimazole (another antibiotic) oral lozenges can be used daily until the condition clears up. Sometimes, *Candida* in the mouth is resistant to topical approaches, or it may extend down the throat into the esophagus. In these cases, a single oral dose of fluconazole or another similar oral antifungal drug may be used. At the corners of the mouth, topical antifungal drugs—nystatin, terbinafine, clotrimazole, miconazole, ketoconazole, or econazole—may be useful. They are generally applied once or twice a day initially and then once or twice a week after the rash has been resolved to prevent recurrences.

The corners of the mouth must be kept clean and dry. It is often useful to eat fruits and vegetables with a fork and to drink juices with a straw to prevent moisture from accumulating at the corners of the mouth.

In the body folds, it is important to control yeast infections because they can lead to secondary bacterial infections and surface breakdown of the skin. The area should be kept clean using a mild soap. After cleansing, the area should be thoroughly patted dry and an antifungal drug should be applied.

In the vaginal area, internal yeast infections are treated with over-the-counter or prescription vaginal creams or vaginal suppositories. These infections often cause a disturbing itch and may be accompanied by a vaginal discharge. Difficult cases may require oral antiyeast therapy with a single dose of fluoconazole or several days of an oral antifungal drug such as itraconazole or ketoconazole.

Cleanse the rectal area with water before using a topical antifungal agent. If stools are liquid or loosely formed, you need to eat more fiber or add bulk-forming agents to your diet.

Candidal infections often come back, so your physician may advise a preventative program of using antifungal powders applied with a cotton ball or periodic application of topical antifungal creams to prevent the infection from returning.

Which bacterial infections might bother you?

Bacteria can cause many different changes in the skin. The infections can involve both the outer layer of skin (epidermis) and the deeper, second layer of skin (dermis). These infections include impetigo, erythrasma, erysipelas, folliculitis, cellulitis, the very rare necrotizing fasciitis and cellulitis, and abscesses. See chapter 14 for more on infections.

Impetigo

Impetigo is a yellow, honeycomb-crusted spot on a red base that is often seen on the face or hands. It may sometimes be associated with blisters. This infection involves the epidermis. It is caused by bacteria called *Staphylococcus aureus* or *Streptococcus*.

Localized impetigo is often successfully treated with antibacterials such as mupirocin (Bactroban) or bacitracin (Baciquent). If multiple spots are present, oral antibiotics are often necessary. People with bacterial infections (as well as their close personal contacts) may be carrying organisms in

their nostrils, groin, or other parts of the body not involved
with the skin rash. Your doctor may want to culture these
areas to be sure further treatment is not necessary.

Erythrasma

This superficial bacterial infection appears as brownish,
itchy patches in moist skin folds, particularly in the genital
and underarm areas. Erythrasma resembles fungal skin
infections, but the lesion borders are not elevated, there are
no satellite lesions, and microscopic preparations do not
show fungal elements. Diagnosis can usually be made by
the appearance, but under ultraviolet light, the patches emit
a characteristic coral-red fluorescence (glow). The condition
often has no symptoms, but it may cause itching or even
breakdown of the skin. If treatment is required, the oral
antibiotic erythromycin is usually effective.

Erysipelas

Deeper infections in the second layer of skin include
erysipelas. Erysipelas usually presents with hot, red, hive-like
spots on one side of the face, but it may spread quickly. This
infection will often make you feel ill with general malaise and
fever. Prompt attention is important, and an emergency visit to
your doctor at the nearest hospital is advised. Treatment usually requires intravenous antibiotics.

Folliculitis

Diabetes appears to increase your likelihood of developing
several common bacterial infections, usually caused by
Staphylococci. Part of the reason is a high rate of coloniza-
tion of the nose with *Staphylococci*, which then shed onto
the skin. These infections often begin in hair follicles and are
thus called *folliculitis*. Larger and deeper infections are
called *furuncles*, which may then progress to carbuncles.
This lesion most often occurs on the back of the neck. These

infections cause red, warm, tender ("sore as a boil") swellings of the skin, sometimes with draining pus. Mild infections may respond to antibiotic therapy alone, but more extensive lesions require surgical drainage.

Cellulitis

Another type of skin infection that appears to be more frequent or severe in people with diabetes is called *cellulitis*, which is a red and tender swelling, often on the feet or legs but occasionally elsewhere. Here, the infection spreads more superficially and is most often caused by *Streptococci*. This infection usually responds promptly (within 36–48 hours) to antibiotic therapy, although it may appear to worsen in the first 24 hours. If the infection does not improve, it is important to reevaluate and look for organisms resistant to the antibiotic you are taking or for a more serious infection, such as a necrotizing fasciitis or cellulitis. Unless these infections are caught in the very early stages, intravenous antibiotics are necessary.

Necrotizing fasciitis and cellulitis

People with diabetes are more susceptible to these potentially life-threatening, subcutaneous (below the skin) soft-tissue infections. Infection causing death of soft tissue is called *necrotizing fasciitis*. Fasciitis means involvement of the skin down to the fascia, the tissue that covers the muscle. *Necrotizing cellulitis* usually involves the muscle as well. Gangrene may also develop, and it usually causes gas in tissues. Necrotizing infections are characterized by their rapid onset and spread, with tissue destruction. Clues to their presence include severe pain, development of blisters, and bleeding into the skin. Your BG level may be higher than normal. Fortunately, these types of infection are uncommon. They are more apt to occur in patients with impaired circulation, after trauma, and in deeper infections, especially of the lower extremities, genital, or rectal areas. A particular form of necrotizing infection that involves the male genitals is called *Fournier's gangrene*. Treatment for these infections must include immediate, aggressive surgical debridement of the necrotic tissue along with broad-spectrum intravenous antibiotics.

Abscesses

An abscess is a confined area containing microorganisms (usually bacteria) and white blood cells (pus). In people with diabetes, these may occur in the area of insulin injections and are often caused by contaminated needles, syringes, or multiple-dose vials. To help prevent this problem, you should clean your injection site and the tops of any multiuse vials.

Which fungal infections should you know about?

Fungal infections are usually caused by one of two types of fungi: dermatophytes or yeasts, such as *Candida*. Infections cause redness, scaling, itching, and sometimes skin breakdown. They are easily treated with antifungal creams and can be prevented by keeping the areas clean and dry and by controlling blood glucose levels.

Fungal infections may appear between your toes, around your groin, under breasts, on the bottoms of your feet, on the palms of your hands, or on and under your nails.

Fungal infections usually start between the fourth and fifth toes because this is where the toes are most tightly compacted. White and softened skin is the first sign of infection that gradually spreads to the other toe web spaces. It can be treated with topical over-the-counter antifungals (clotrimazole, miconazole) twice a day. Dry between your toes very well after bathing and then apply the topical antifungal. When the infection clears, use an antifungal powder daily to keep the toe webs dry.

Fungal infections of the groin are more common in men. They involve the inner thighs, with a red active scaly area and central clearing, and spare the scrotum. Use topical antifungals once or twice a day for active infection and antifungal powder to help prevent recurrences. Boxer shorts can help keep the area dry. Tight-fitting clothing, overweight, and athletic activities with a lot of sweating and friction lead to frequent recurrences.

Another fungal infection involves the soles of your feet and palms of your hands. A dry powdery scale that often starts in a small area gradually spreads to the entire sole or palm surface. The dry skin often spreads around the sides of the feet, which is referred to as "moccasin-type" changes. If topical antifungal cream is not successful, you may need a short course of oral antifungal agents (terbinafine, itraconazole).

The most cosmetically disturbing fungal infection involves your fingernails and toenails. The nails become thick and yellow. This infection is most common in the large toenails but can spread to the other nails of the feet or hands (chapter 14).

Do diabetes medications affect your skin?

Yes. The diabetes pills called sulfonylureas can cause minor changes in your skin, and so can insulin.

Sulfonylureas

Skin rashes are the most common side effect in the first few months of therapy and are seen in 1–5% of cases. The rash often looks like measles. Be careful in the sun. Hives and an allergic reaction can occur on sun-exposed skin. The measles-like rash may disappear on its own even if you continue taking the medication, but other kinds of rashes would require you to stop taking this medication.

Any alcohol that you drink may interact with chlor-propamide and cause flushing of your whole body and especially your face. Skin reactions and flushing are uncommon with the newer second-generation sulfonylureas. If you have a reaction to oral sulfonylurea drugs, there is approximately a 20% chance of your reacting to a number of related chemicals, including

- permanent hair dye (paraphenylenediamine)
- a component of sun screens called PABA (para-aminobenzoic acid)
- local anesthetic creams (benzocaine)
- some diuretic pills (hydrochlorothiazide)
- sulfonamide antibiotics

Insulin

Skin reactions to insulin are less common with newer, purer forms of insulin. Local reactions may start with burning at the injection site, followed by a hivelike reaction that may fade over hours to days. Skin reactions may be immediate or delayed. Generalized hives and even respiratory or circulatory collapse due to insulin allergy are extremely rare.

Delayed reactions at insulin injection sites include changes in the fat under the skin. The fat may be decreased, causing little indentations on the surface (lipoatrophy), but this complication is much less common with newer purified insulins. If an insulin site is used repeatedly for years, the fat may actually increase in size, causing an elevated bump (hypertrophy). This is a very common condition, and repeatedly injecting into this area is a common cause of brittle diabetes. Darkening or thickening of the skin may also be seen at insulin injection sites.

R. Gary Sibbald, MD, contributed to this chapter.

16

Psychosocial Complications

Introduction

Diabetes can be a hell of a disease. Even if your blood glucose control is good and you haven't developed any long-term complications, living with diabetes is no fun. There are no vacations: diabetes is a 24-hour-a-day, 365-day-a-year proposition. Add to that the fact that diabetes affects every aspect of your life, forces you to stick yourself countless times a day, and makes you deprive yourself of foods you crave. And that's not all. If you succeed in keeping your blood glucose levels close to normal, your risk of going too low (hypoglycemia) goes up, and often so does your weight. To top it off, you must live with the fact that there are no guarantees when it comes to diabetes. You can do everything right and still get a blood glucose reading you can't explain.

It's no wonder that a condition we call *diabetes overwhelmus* is so common. Many people are simply overwhelmed by the daily demands of their diabetes treatment. Diabetes overwhelmus may not be an official term, but it is a serious problem. People who suffer from it tell us they are often caught in a negative spiral. Feeling overwhelmed, they find it terribly hard to maintain good self-care, which leads to worsened blood glucose control, which makes their diabetes overwhelmus even worse.

In this chapter, we tell you about the various forms diabetes overwhelmus can take, how common each one is among people with diabetes, and how you can tell whether you are suffering from any of them. You need to know what you and your health care providers can do to prevent, detect, and treat diabetes overwhelmus

Is there a quick way for you to check your psychological condition?

Everyone gets down in the dumps from time to time, even if they don't have diabetes. Having diabetes only makes it more likely that you will have some down times. If your blue periods are rare, pass quickly, and don't interfere much with your ability to take good care of yourself, you probably don't need the information in this chapter. If, on the other hand, emotional struggles are a regular part of your life with diabetes, read on.

What kind of psychological problems come with diabetes?

Diabetes-related psychological problems fall into two broad categories—coping difficulties and psychological disorders. Coping difficulties are more common, and psychological disorders are more serious. Let's talk about the more common problems first.

Are you feeling discouraged?

You don't need to have a psychological disorder like clinical depression to feel demoralized about living with diabetes. The unending demands can make you feel that. You are especially likely to feel discouraged when you experience one of the predictable "crises" of diabetes. These crises include finding out you have diabetes, having to change your treatment regimen (for example, going from diabetes pills to insulin), and developing a complication (eye, kidney, or heart disease, for example). When any of these events occur, you are likely to feel discouraged and even helpless. These reactions are normal and natural. There are things you can do to dramatically improve the situation. Complications can be treated and some can even be reversed.

What fears come with diabetes?

Fear can be immobilizing. For example, many people fear diabetes complications so much they try to manage their fear by denying that anything can happen to them. But that only prevents them from doing the things that would reduce their risk of getting complications!

Fear may also show up in other areas of diabetes management. Some people fear sticking themselves to check BG or to give themselves insulin. Working closely with your health care provider, a diabetes educator, or a mental health professional familiar with diabetes can help you overcome fears like these.

If you take insulin, fear of hypoglycemia can keep you from trying for close-to-normal blood glucose levels (see chapter 2).

You may also have fears that people will treat you differently because you have diabetes. Whom should you tell about your diabetes, and what should you tell them? If you take insulin, it's important to let people you spend lots of time with know that you have diabetes. Otherwise, they may misunderstand why you carry injection equipment, need to eat at certain times, and what to do when your blood glucose is low.

Diabetes is nothing to be ashamed of; it is part of you. The closer you are to someone, the more important it is that they know about you. People generally respond if you tell them what you need; for example, "I need something to eat right now because I have diabetes."

You may fear that having diabetes will affect your ability to get and keep a job. While a few careers are closed to people who have diabetes or those who take insulin, most job-related discrimination based on the fact that you have diabetes is against the law. If you experience discrimination that you feel is illegal, contact a local ADA office. The ADA cannot give legal advice, but they may be able to advise you of existing remedies pertaining to your situation. In general, the Americans with Disabilities Act prevents people from discriminating against you because of your diabetes.

Some parents who have children with diabetes worry about the child's care at school. Education for parents, teachers, and classmates can help. One option is to obtain an excellent film for elementary school children called "The School Day and Diabetes Basics for Teachers and Staff K-4." The film is available by writing to the Biomedical Communications Center for Educational Television, P.O. Box 19230, Southern Illinois University, Springfield, IL 62749. You can also contact the ADA at 1-800-DIABETES or check the Wizdom section of the ADA web site (www.diabetes.org/wizdom).

How can you cope with eating problems?

People often eat not because they are hungry but to make themselves feel better. This can be unhealthy for anyone, but especially for people with diabetes. You might feel guilty about it. Many people feel guilty and discouraged by the way they eat. Unfortunately, these feelings often make matters worse, sapping the energy you need to get back on track. When you fall off the wagon (and everyone does), try to get right back on. One doughnut, or even several of them, is not going to ruin a diet unless you become discouraged and give up.

Being too controlled about what foods you eat can be a problem. Some people measure every bite they eat and deny themselves even the smallest amount of "forbidden foods." This approach works for some people but not many. For most people, this leads to frustration and uncontrolled eating. You need to find an approach that you can live with over the long run rather than cycling back and forth between overcontrolled and undercontrolled eating.

Where can you get help for day-to-day diabetes problems?

If you are feeling overwhelmed by the demands of managing your diabetes, talk to your health care provider about ways to make your treatment plan less demanding. It might seem like wishful thinking but there's almost always a way to make diabetes self-care a little easier. It would probably help to join a diabetes support group and talk with people who know what you are going through. Discussing treatments with them may help you find other ways to make your diabetes management easier.

Staying current about the latest developments in diabetes research and treatment can also help. The ADA publishes a wonderful magazine called *Diabetes Forecast*, which you can get by joining ADA—call 1-800-806-7801. Books on diabetes, available from ADA and in bookstores, are another excellent source of ideas. This information can help you identify changes you could make in your diabetes self-care, and you can talk with your health care provider about them.

Where can you get help learning about and practicing self-care skills?

The key to living well with diabetes is putting knowledge into action. Think about one of your self-care skills that isn't as sharp as you'd like it to be. How could you improve this skill? Would working with your health care provider help? Do you need a referral for help with your meal plan, exercise program, or glucose checking technique? Consider going to a diabetes education program where you can learn about all of the latest approaches to good care. Be sure the program focuses on self-care *skills* and not on information alone. More and more insurance companies are realizing the value of diabetes education programs—they help you prevent serious complications and improve your day-to-day health—and your program may be covered by your health insurance.

Another source of help is diabetes counseling from a behavioral specialist (mental health counselor, psychologist, or social worker) or a behaviorally trained diabetes educator. These professionals can help you identify your personal barriers or "sticking points." We have found that being very specific is crucial to success in this process. The more specifically a sticking point is defined, the easier it is to solve. While many people might say that difficulty eating right is their sticking point; one man defined his problem more specifically, which made it much easier to solve. He said that he had an overpowering desire to snack between dinner and bedtime.

Once the specific sticking point is identified, the counselor can help you problem solve, paying attention to any approaches you may have used successfully in the past. This process can help you learn new ways to cope better with diabetes. Good problem-solving skills can be developed through practice, like any other skill. You can become your own diabetes counselor; in fact, there's no one in the world more qualified for the job.

People with diabetes cope better when they get practical and emotional support from family and friends. If you think you are getting less support than you need, try to talk to those whose help you need. Be calm, don't bring up the subject when you are upset. Do not talk about how the other person failed you in the past. Accentuate the positive. Tell the person how he or she helped you in the past, and that what you are looking for is more of the same. If this approach doesn't work for you, consider making an appointment with your health care provider for yourself and your support person. You could ask the person to attend a diabetes support group meeting or a diabetes education class with you. These can all be good ways for you to help those who care about you be more helpful. It's easier for everyone to cope when they have a little help.

What psychological disorders are common among people with diabetes?

Psychological disorders are basically extreme versions of the coping problems many people with diabetes have. Some psychological problems to watch for are depression, anxiety disorder, and eating disorders. People with diabetes are more likely to have these problems, and they tend to last longer, feel worse, and recur more often. In addition, having a psychological disorder makes diabetes management much more difficult.

What are the symptoms of depression?

Distinguishing between temporarily feeling blue and being truly depressed can be tricky, but we hope the signs and symptoms described below will help you decide which side of the line you are on.

Depression is probably the most common psychological disorder among people with diabetes. When most people say they are depressed, they don't use the term in the clinical sense. They are generally talking about feeling sad and dragged out emotionally in the way almost everyone does from time to time. These feelings come and go, usually in a couple of hours or a couple of days. Clinical depression is not like that; it takes you way down and keeps you there a long time. Clinical depression is diagnosed when a person has five or more specific symptoms for at least 2 weeks. Look at the symptoms in Table 16-1. If you have had either of the first two symptoms and at least four of the other listed symptoms for at least two weeks, you may be suffering from clinical depression. A glance at this table makes it clear that depression really is different from a case of the blues.

Table 16-1. Signs of Clinical Depression

1. Depressed mood (feeling sad or empty) most of the day nearly every day

2. Markedly diminished interest or pleasure in all, or almost all, activities most of the day nearly every day

3. Significant weight loss when not dieting, weight gain (for example, a change of more than 5% of body weight in a month), or decrease or increase in appetite nearly every day

4. Trouble sleeping or sleeping too much nearly every day

5. Feeling really agitated or physically sluggish nearly every day

6. Fatigue or loss of energy nearly every day

7. Feeling worthless or excessively or inappropriately guilty nearly every day

8. Diminished ability to think or concentrate, or indecisiveness, nearly every day

9. Recurrent thoughts of death (not just fear of dying), recurrent thoughts of suicide, a suicide attempt, or a specific plan to commit suicide

Too many people with diabetes who are depressed aren't getting the treatment they need. That's really too bad, because there are effective treatments. Don't be afraid to talk to your health care provider if you think you might be depressed. Effective treatment not only improves your quality of life, but studies show that it could also dramatically improve your blood glucose control as well.

What works to relieve depression?

If you feel that you might be depressed, you should talk to your health care provider. First, describe your symptoms to be sure he or she knows what's going on. Then talk about treatment options. In our experience, the best treatment for depression combines counseling and medication.

How can you find a counselor who fits your needs?

We know that getting into counseling can be a big step. Maybe you are a private person, and the idea of talking about your problems with someone you don't know might not sit right for you. You might not believe in counseling. Naturally, you are the only one who can decide if counseling is for you, but we strongly encourage you to consider this option. Counseling does work.

Cognitive-behavioral therapy (CBT), which focuses on current problems and how to deal with them, is especially effective in treating diabetes-related psychological problems, so try to find a therapist who specializes in this approach. In one study of people with diabetes who were depressed, some people got 8 sessions of CBT and others got 8 sessions of diabetes education. After the sessions were done, people in the CBT group were much more likely to have recovered from their depression, and they had much bigger improvements in blood glucose control.

Try to find a counselor who has experience working with people who have diabetes. Unfortunately, counselors who specialize in treating people with diabetes are rare. If you can't find one, look for one who is willing to learn, through information you or your diabetes health provider can offer. You could also call the ADA at 1-800-342-2383 (1-800-DIABETES) or the American Association of Diabetes Educators (AADE) at 1-800-338-3633. They can provide the names of diabetes educators in your area who specialize in mental health services.

What medicines are used to treat depression?

Medications can be a big help in treating depression, but they are most effective when used in combination with counseling. Only a physician can tell whether medications would help you and prescribe the right one(s) for you.

Most antidepressants on the market today fall into one of two classes. The first class is *tricyclic antidepressants* and includes such drugs as Elavil (amitriptyline), Tofranil (imipramine), Sinequan (doxepin), and Pamelor (nortripty-line). Tricyclic antidepressants are prescribed less often than in the past. Tricyclics may have side effects, including dry mouth, sleepiness, increased appetite and weight gain, and sexual dysfunction. Although most people don't experience these side effects, some of them can be especially troublesome for people with diabetes.

A newer class of antidepressants is the *selective serotonin reuptake inhibitors* (SSRIs). Drugs in this class include Prozac (fluoxetine), Paxil (paroxetine), Zoloft (sertraline), Serzone (nefazodone), and Effexor (venlafaxine). These medications don't seem to make people as sleepy. In addition, they actually tend to decrease appetite and lead to weight loss in some people. This is called a *benign side-effect profile*. It helps explain why so many prescriptions are being written for this class of antidepressants. SSRIs do cause gastrointestinal distress, sexual problems, or over-stimulation in some people.

If you start taking any antidepressant medication, it's important to keep in mind that the drug usually takes a couple of weeks or longer to begin producing its full beneficial effect. Unfortunately, the side effects begin much earlier (if you are going to experience any at all), and then they generally become less troublesome. So there may be a period of days or weeks after you begin taking an antidepressant when the only real effect you get will be a negative one. Be sure to tell the physician who prescribed the medication about both the benefits and side effects you are experiencing.

Both classes of antidepressant medication have been shown to relieve depression in people with diabetes, and relieving depression seems to be associated with a significant improvement in blood glucose control. So, treating depression with counseling, medication, or a combination of the two, can help improve your physical and emotional health.

What is anxiety disorder?

Anxiety disorder is another serious psychological problem, found to be much more common among people who have diabetes than it is among the general population. Again, it's important to distinguish between normal anxiety and a diagnosable disorder. Everyone worries about things sometimes. Some of these worries may be diabetes related; others may not be. Worrying about your blood sugars or about complications is normal, as is worrying about your job or your family.

A clinical anxiety disorder is different. When you have a clinical anxiety disorder, the worries are so intense, so uncomfortable, and so long lasting that they interfere with your ability to function at work, at home, and in other important areas of your life.

What are the symptoms of anxiety disorder?

You are probably suffering from a clinical anxiety disorder if you have been uncontrollably anxious for at least six months about a number of events or activities (such as work or school performance or your diabetes management) **and** during that period you had at least three of the symptoms listed in Table 16-2 for more days than you did not.

Table 16-2. Signs of Anxiety Disorder

1. Restlessness or feeling keyed up or on edge
2. Being easily fatigued
3. Difficulty concentrating or mind going blank
4. Irritability
5. Muscle tension
6. Sleep disturbance (difficulty falling or staying asleep, or restless, unsatisfying sleep)

You probably noticed that some of these symptoms are identical to those of clinical depression. There is an overlap, because some psychological problems share similar symptoms, and because some people suffer from more than one disorder. This makes an important point: If you have any signs of a clinical psychological disorder, get help. You don't need to diagnose yourself to know that you need help.

Are there treatments for anxiety disorders?

Counseling can help you find ways to cope better with your fears. If you are suffering from anxiety disorder, there are also medications that might help. Commonly prescribed anti-anxiety drugs include Ativan (lorazepam), BuSpar (buspirone), Serax (oxazepam), Tranxene (clorazepate), and Xanax (alprazolam).

Please keep in mind that the effectiveness of all mood-altering drugs is an individual matter. Different medications, even those closely related chemically, seem to affect different people differently. So you may need to try more than one medication before you find the right one for you.

What are eating disorders?

Again, it is important to distinguish between normal behavior and behavior that indicates a problem. Spending a lot of time thinking about what you eat and carefully managing your eating are signs you are taking good care of your diabetes. Many people are concerned with eating and weight even if they don't have diabetes. Unfortunately, when these tendencies are combined, the result can be a full-blown eating disorder.

Eating disorders come in two forms. The first, which involves eating very, very little food often combined with extreme levels of exercise, is called *anorexia nervosa*. The other, which involves binge eating followed by purging, usually in the form of vomiting or the use of diuretics or laxatives, is called *bulimia nervosa*. It should come as no surprise that having either type of eating disorder enormously complicates diabetes care. In fact, there is no way you can effectively manage your diabetes if you have an active eating disorder.

How can you tell if you have an eating disorder?

Many people want to be thin (and feel disappointed if they are not), exercise to manage weight and stay fit, and occasionally eat more than they should. It is normal to eat prunes or use other approaches for occasional constipation and to use diuretics, when your doctor prescribes them, to treat fluid retention or high blood pressure. It is normal to adjust insulin doses to maintain good blood glucose control. It is not normal to engage in extreme forms of these behaviors. If you (or someone you care about) have any of the signs listed in Table 16-3, you may have an eating disorder.

Table 16-3. Signs of Eating Disorder

1. Weigh less than 85% of normal for your height, body frame, and age
2. Have an intense fear of gaining weight or becoming fat, even though you are underweight
3. See yourself as fat when others say you are too thin
4. Exercise far more than is necessary to stay fit
5. Miss at least three consecutive menstrual cycles
6. Deny the seriousness of your low body weight
7. Binge eat (eat very large amounts of food at a single sitting), at least twice a week for 3 months
8. Feel you can't stop eating or control what or how much you are eating
9. Vomit food you have eaten, or use diuretics, laxatives, enemas, or other medications to lose weight or prevent weight gain
10. Deliberately take less insulin than you need to maintain good blood glucose control with the conscious intent of managing your weight by passing some of the calories you consume as glucose in urine

What does insulin manipulation have to do with eating disorders?

Insulin manipulation is a frightening eating-disordered behavior unique to people with diabetes. This behavior is horrifyingly common. Some researchers estimate that as many as 50% of all young women frequently take less insulin than they need in an effort to control their weight. Decreasing the insulin leads to high blood glucose and loss of sugar (calories) and water in the urine. This causes weight loss but at a terrible price. Manipulating insulin doses to control or lose weight and other eating disorder behaviors can lead to DKA and hospitalization and raise the risk of developing complications.

Are there treatments for eating disorders?

People who have eating disorders feel they must control their eating, and they are usually terrified at the prospect of giving up this control. Most don't want anyone to know they have an eating disorder, because they feel deeply ashamed. You may believe no one can understand what you are going through or help you, but that's not true. You need a mental health professional who treats people with eating disorders, and hopefully, knows something about diabetes.

No medications are currently available that have been proven to be effective in treating eating disorders, though some researchers have reported success treating people with certain SSRI antidepressants. As we have said, the most effective treatment for eating disorders is intensive psychotherapy. So, if you are suffering from an eating disorder, or if you suspect that you might be, please get help.

What is the last word?

In fact, getting help is the right thing to do no matter what form of diabetes overwhelmus you have. If you are feeling stressed for any reason, that stress will affect your physical and emotional health. Fortunately, there are ways to relieve stress. The right stress-reduction recipe for you depends on the source of your stress—whether it is depression, lack of support from family, or difficulty fitting diabetes care into day-to-day life. Help may come in the form of medication, a support group, or nutritional counseling. Talk to your health care provider to find the help you need. That can make the whole world seem brighter—and diabetes management a little less daunting.

This chapter was written by Richard R. Rubin, PhD, CDE, and Mark Peyrot, PhD.

17

Men's Sexual Health

Case study

JG is a 32-year-old married man who came to his family practitioner with complaints of progressive loss of the ability to get and maintain an erection. He has had type 1 diabetes for 15 years and has good blood glucose control. In the past 3 years, he has developed some mild neuropathy in both his feet that comes and goes. Although he has maintained near-normal blood glucose levels in recent years, his previous history shows wide swings in glucose levels.

JG first noticed difficulty in maintaining an erection with some decrease in observed morning erections. Over the past 6 months, as neuropathy in his feet became more persistent, he noticed a decrease in the amount of ejaculate, but his feeling of orgasm continued. During the same time, his erectile function continued to decline, and, although he reports occasional partial morning erections, he has no erections satisfactory for sexual activity. JG was referred to his urologist for evaluation and treatment of his erectile dysfunction and ejaculatory changes.

Introduction

Male erectile dysfunction, or impotence, may be defined as an inability to have and maintain an erection rigid enough for sexual intercourse. It has been estimated that more than 18 million American men suffer from erectile dysfunction (ED). It is three times more common in men with diabetes in any age-group. The Massachusetts Male Aging Study (MMAS), the first large-scale study on sexual dysfunction of a general population, evaluated 1,709 randomly chosen men from the Boston suburbs. Of these men, 1,290 (75.5%) completed questionnaires concerning their sexual function. It may surprise you that more than half (52%) of these healthy middle-aged men complained of erectile dysfunction. The study showed that the likelihood of any man having ED increases with age.

The MMAS also reviewed impotence in middle-aged men with diabetes. This and other studies show that diabetes in men more than 40 years old is associated with increasing erectile dysfunction. In this group as a whole, impotence was 11% more common than in the nondiabetic group.

Nonetheless, there is hope. There are ways to diminish your risks and to improve your overall health, which will improve your libido (interest in sex) and enjoyment.

Are there ways of predicting who will have ED?

In the MMAS, the factors that researchers found helpful in predicting who would have some degree of impotence included alcohol intake, level of blood glucose control, and whether the man had intermittent claudication (pain in the legs while walking, a sign of vascular disease in the legs), retinopathy, or neuropathy (nerve damage).

What puts you at risk for developing ED?

ED can be caused by physical conditions, injury, or emotional or psychological conditions or as a side effect of medications that you are taking. It can be caused by drugs such as alcohol or marijuana.

Medical problems associated with ED include heart disease, hypertension, and high cholesterol. This is no surprise, because all of these abnormalities relate to circulation. And your risk of developing circulation problems is intensified by cigarette smoking. Having poor blood glucose control for long periods of time also puts you at risk for developing ED. JG had wide swings in blood glucose levels for several years and was suffering from peripheral neuropathy in his feet as a result. His problems achieving an erection could be due to nerve damage, which can result from poor glucose control.

Psychological risk factors associated with impotence in all men include depression, anger, and low self-esteem. These are as powerful as any physical factor and often contribute to the problem even if they are not the main cause. JG is a young man and is having emotional difficulty accepting his loss of sexual function.

The drugs you take for other conditions can also put you at risk for ED. These drugs include blood pressure drugs such as beta blockers and diuretics, some antidepressants, and some stomach ulcer medications. Over-the-counter medications can also cause problems, as can recreational drugs such as alcohol and marijuana. Discuss with your health care provider whether any medication that you are taking is causing or adding to your experience of ED (Table 17-1). On rare occasions, low levels of testosterone will put you at risk.

How does an erection normally occur?

The complex process that results in an erection includes emotions, hormones, blood circulation, and nerves. Nerve pathways to and from the brain can initiate (or inhibit) your erectile response. Seeing or imagining things that are sexually exciting and touching or having your penis touched activate these signals from the brain. There are changes in blood circulation that allow more blood to flow into and be "dammed up"

Table 17-1. Medications Associated with Male Erectile Dysfunction

Anti-Hypertensive (High blood pressure)	1. Diuretics 2. Vasodilators 3. Central sympatholytics 4. Ganglion blockers 5. Beta blockers 6. ACE inhibitors 7. Calcium-channel blockers
Antiandrogens (testosterone)	1. Estrogens 2. Luteinizing-hormone–releasing hormone agonists
Anticholinergics	1. Atropine 2. Propantheline 3. Diphydramine
Antidepressants	1. Tricydines 2. Monoamine oxidase inhibitors 3. Serotonin re-uptake inhibitors
Antianxiety Drugs	1. Benzodiazepines 2. Phenothiazines 3. Butyrophenones
Miscellaneous	1. Alcohol 2. Marijuana 3. Cocaine 4. Barbiturates 5. Nicotine 6. Cimetidine 7. Clofibrate 8. Digoxin 9. Indomethacin

in the penis. This forms the rigid structure of an erection. Both the inflow and the damming of the blood are necessary for the erection to occur and be maintained. This is all done under the influence of nerves that work automatically—the autonomic nerves.

What part do hormones play in the erection process?

Male hormone, or testosterone, is essential for erectile function. Also, hormones in the central nervous system influence sexual activity by increasing libido and sexual behavior. If you are less and less interested in sex, you might have low male hormone levels, but this condition is relatively uncommon. If you do need testosterone replacement, your health care provider can determine why it is low and can give you testosterone in one of several forms.

What can cause ED in a man with diabetes?

There can be many causes. It may be a result of peripheral neuropathy (nerve damage), atherosclerosis (clogged arteries), or decreased testosterone levels. ED can be caused by prescription medications for high blood pressure, such as beta blockers and diuretics, for depression, for ulcers, or to prevent vomiting. It can be caused or made worse by psychological factors. It can be caused by injury. The most common physical causes of ED with diabetes are blood vessel disease with decreased circulation and nerve damage. Both of these conditions are complications of diabetes. Add to these health problems the stress of worries and fears about aging, diabetes, complications, and sexual performance and you have the formula for ED.

What is ejaculatory dysfunction?

Peripheral neuropathy appears to be responsible for the ejaculatory abnormalities frequently encountered in as many as 32% of men with diabetes. The most common of these dysfunctions is the one JG encountered, a decrease in the amount of ejaculate (retrograde ejaculation). Retrograde ejaculation is ejaculation backward into the bladder. It is caused by nerve dysfunction and can occasionally be overcome by the use of certain drugs. If you suspect that this is your problem, you should consult a urologist or your primary health care provider.

How is ED diagnosed?

JG's appointment with his health care provider began with a full history, complete physical examination, and appropriate laboratory tests. Sometimes, male erectile dysfunction may be the first indication of diabetes or vascular disease.

JG's initial history included the date when his erectile dysfunction began (6 months earlier) and the presence or absence of previous erectile function (it had never happened before). JG's provider asked whether his erectile dysfunction was accompanied by ejaculatory dysfunction, diminished interest in sex, or failure to reach orgasm. To determine the possible causes, your provider needs to know about the last episode of successful sexual intercourse, how often erectile problems occur, whether you have nighttime and morning erections or erections during masturbation, and whether you have ED only with a certain partner or situation.

How are psychological causes of ED diagnosed?

Men with psychological ED will still have morning, nighttime, and self-stimulated erections. The onset of ED in these men is often sudden and may be related to a specific life event. If this is the case, your provider would take a more detailed psycho-sexual history exploring the sources of anxiety, relationship problems, stress, and possible depression.

ED from physical causes is more often a gradual loss of rigidity with decreases in morning and nighttime erections, much like JG's experience.

What other questions will your health care provider ask?

Your provider will ask about any medications you are taking. Sexual dysfunction is frequently caused by high blood pressure medications (Table 17-1). Antidepressant medications may allow you to maintain an erection but may make ejaculation more difficult. Your provider will ask whether you drink alcohol or smoke and how often.

What happens during your physical examination?

Your physical examination should include the external genitalia, prostate, and hair distribution on the feet and legs. You'll also have your blood pressure, cardiac status, and legs and feet checked to see whether circulation problems are contributing to sexual dysfunction.

What laboratory tests need to be done?

Laboratory tests must include a urine analysis and blood glucose level. Elevated blood glucose in a patient with ED are sometimes how his diabetes is first diagnosed. Blood levels of testosterone and other hormone studies may be important in identifying specific causes for organic (physical) ED.

How is ED treated?

ED can be treated in several ways, depending on whether it is brought on by physical or emotional causes. There are both oral and injection drugs, physical devices, and surgical implants. You and your health care provider will choose a treatment based on the physical and psychological factors affecting your condition.

What if your testosterone levels are too low?

It is unusual that you would need testosterone replacement. However, if your blood tests indicate it, there are a couple of ways—by injection or skin patches. Oral tablets are seldom used because they don't work as well as the patch and may be toxic to your liver.

Normal testosterone concentrations vary throughout the day, with the highest levels appearing early in the morning and the lowest around midnight. Testosterone injected into the muscles doesn't do this. It produces a very high initial concentration that falls to a level below normal before the next injection. So a patch was developed.

Testosterone skin patches can be applied over muscles or on the scrotum. The treatment requires daily application of patches, which produces blood levels of testosterone similar to normal levels. Patients report improved energy level, mood, strength, libido and sexual function, and nighttime erections. The patch can cause skin irritation and itching, but these side effects are usually temporary and can be treated with topical agents.

Are there pills for ED?

Yohimbine (Aphrodyne), an oral medication for ED, comes from the bark of the yohimbe tree and has been used for more than a century as an aphrodisiac (a substance thought to enhance sexual desire). Studies in men with psychologically caused ED have demonstrated a positive response in 31% of men taking yohimbine. There have been no clinical trials of this drug only in men with diabetes, mainly because men with diabetes do not complain of ED until it is beyond the stage where yohimbine will help. Yohimbine tends to help patients who still have erections but have a rigidity problem; most patients with diabetes have lost both when they come for treatment. Penile rings seem to work almost as well, if not better, than yohimbine for this problem or can be used in combination with it. You can use a penis ring with the medicated urethral system for erection (MUSE, discussed below) as well, if you achieve better results that way.

One of the most talked about pills is sildenafil (Viagra), which stimulates and maintains erectile function. Its affect appears to be most significant when taken 30–60 minutes before intercourse. Although studies specific to diabetic men have not been performed for sildenafil, it works well on a wide variety of causes of male ED.

Men who have had a heart attack or stroke in the past six months or with blood pressure below 90/50 or higher than 170/110, or with unstable angina should only use Viagra with caution. If any erection lasts for longer than 4 hours, get emergency treatment.

What about injection treatments for ED?

A variety of drugs are available, have been used throughout the world, and have helped many diabetic men with chronic ED. Unless you have severe vascular disease, injection therapy appears to be one of the most effective methods for restoring potency. Side effects include an increase in thickened tissue, prolonged erection, and pain.

What do you need to learn about using these drugs?

The first time you use the drug should be in a clinic to learn the proper technique and to monitor the effectiveness of the drug and any side effects, such as prolonged erection. The first dose is low, to demonstrate the injection technique. Doses are increased until you get a good-quality erection that does not last too long.

You will be shown how to fill the syringe. An area at the side of the penis is chosen, and the skin is cleansed with alcohol. Then, the skin is held tight, and the needle is placed in the corpus cavernosum (erectile tissue) at the base of the penis. This can be performed on either side, avoiding superficial veins. If the erection is inadequate, an increased dose is used with the next demonstration, 24–48 hours later.

Are there treatments for ED that don't use injections?

There is a method called the *medicated urethral system for erection* (MUSE). Alprostadil (prostaglandin E_1) is a tiny suppository that is inserted painlessly with an applicator into the opening at the end of the penis. This system works much like injection therapy but without a needle and is effective for most users. Or you may want to try sildenafil (Viagra), an oral medication you take 30–60 minutes before intercourse. It has been shown to be effective for a large majority of users.

What are the side effects of these other systems?

Side effects of the MUSE system include low blood pressure in a few patients and pain in as many as one-third of patients. Viagra does not seem to interact with the medications you might be taking such as ACE inhibitors or antidepressants. A few users report headaches, flushing, or vision changes such as a color tinge or fuzziness.

What are vacuum constriction devices?

The vacuum device has a long, clear plastic tube (vacuum chamber), pump, and constriction band, which is applied to the base of the penis after erection is achieved. The vacuum chamber is attached to a vacuum pump on one end and open on the other. This open end is placed over the penis, and a seal is obtained at the base with lubricant jelly. The pump mechanism creates a vacuum of approximately 100 mmHg, pulling blood into the penis and creating an erection. Once the erection has become complete, an elastic ring is moved from the tube around the base of the penis to prevent blood from flowing back out of the penis. These devices are used by many patients with diabetes or vascular disease or after radical surgery. Satisfaction achieved is about the same as from an erection achieved by other methods.

Are there any side effects from use of the vacuum device?

Side effects from the vacuum device include feeling cold and numb during erection, with difficulty ejaculating because of the ring. Some patients have difficulty obtaining orgasm as a result of this feeling. Changes in penile skin as well as curvature have been reported from frequent use of the vacuum device. The ring can cause tissue damage. Despite these problems, patient and partner satisfaction appear to be satisfactory in many studies.

Are penile rings used alone?

A penile ring is an elastic band that is placed at the base of the erect penis to keep blood in it (maintaining the erection) during intercourse. Rings may be used alone or in combination with the vacuum device, injections, or MUSE system.

What about surgical implants?

This therapy is not popular and would only be chosen by men who are not satisfied with the other methods. All implants provide rigidity and size to the penis and are enough like a normal erection to permit intercourse. How soft they become between uses, however, varies with the type of device. The prosthetic devices are usable within 4–6 weeks of surgical implantation.

What are the side effects of surgical penile implants?

Infection occurs in about 3% of cases. Higher infection rates have been reported in patients with diabetes. Other complications include breaking or leaking of the fluid in the prosthesis, pain, reduced penile length, and reduced sensation. These are rare but serious enough to concern you, your partner, and your surgeon.

Is there a way to prevent ED?

Do what you can to avoid the one-two punch of poor circulation and nerve damage—maintain good blood glucose, good blood pressure, and good cholesterol levels. Stop smoking. Exercise. Ask your doctor about the side effects of any medications that you have to take.

If you have psychological problems, or suspect that these may be at least in part the cause of your ED, please see a mental health counselor for help solving your problems.

Culley C. Carson, MD, contributed to this chapter.

18

Women's Sexual Health

Case study

LO, a 46-year-old woman diagnosed with type 2 diabetes
5 years ago, has always maintained good glucose control. She
and her husband have been married 20 years and have three
children. Through most of their marriage, they have enjoyed
an active sex life. Lately, however, LO no longer initiates sex
and finds ways to avoid it. Even when she feels emotionally
aroused, she takes a long time to feel physically aroused and
then experiences discomfort during intercourse. As a first step,
the doctor suggests an over-the-counter vaginal lubricant and
that she talk to her husband about what she has been
experiencing.

Case study

Mrs. B, a 36 year old with type 1 diabetes for 27 years, came
to her physician to plan a pregnancy. She had high blood
pressure and protein in her urine. She had high blood glucose
levels and an A1C level of 9.8% (normal range is up to 6).
Her insulin therapy consisted of two insulin injections a day.

Mrs. B's blood pressure and glucose levels needed to
come down before she got pregnant, and the protein in her
urine was too high. Her physician was also concerned about
retinopathy. She was referred to an ophthalmologist for laser

therapy. Her retinas were then in good shape for the pregnancy. A nephrologist placed Mrs. B on blood pressure lowering drugs considered safe for pregnancy. Her health care team helped her with a program of diet, exercise, and medication to bring her blood glucose levels close to normal with an insulin pump and BG monitoring 6 to 8 times a day.

After 6 months, her A1C was in the normal range, and her blood pressure was less than 130/80 mmHg. Mrs. B was given the "go-ahead" to become pregnant. During the pregnancy, her blood pressure, blood glucose levels, and health status all remained good. She delivered a healthy, 7-pound baby boy.

Introduction

Some women define sexuality as the ability to bear children. This definition tends to devalue the whole woman. Sexuality is as important to a woman in her 60s as it is to a woman in her 30s. Women with diabetes can have a healthy and sexually fulfilling life.

What sexual problems can happen to any woman?

It may help to divide sexual problems into two categories: sexual difficulties and sexual dysfunction.

Sexual difficulties

Sexual difficulties are problems in the communication between two people that impact their sexual activity. Generally, these difficulties are a result of lack of knowledge of each other's sexual needs and preferences. They do not or cannot tell each other what they want. A woman will complain that her partner wants sex too often or not often enough, that he does not engage in enough foreplay, or that there is no affectionate closeness after intercourse. She may feel unattracted to her partner, dislike his habits or sexual practices, or be unable to relax with him in sexual play.

Sexual dysfunctions

Sexual dysfunctions are physical problems. Human sexual response normally consists of four events: desire, arousal, orgasm, and satisfaction. Different physiological processes are involved in each phase, so you may have difficulty in one phase but not the others.

Desire is defined for both sexes as the motivation or wish to have a sexual experience. It frequently is a response to an external cue such as an erotic picture or genital pressure. This is an activity that begins in the brain and depends on a certain blood level of hormones. Degree of desire, however, is not dependent on levels of hormones.

Arousal is the emotional and physiological response to mental or tactile erotic stimulation and is expressed both as a feeling of excitement and as an accumulation of blood in the genital area. It is demonstrated by vaginal lubrication.

Orgasm, primarily orchestrated by the nervous system, is characterized by a series of rhythmic contractions of the muscles of the internal reproductive structures and vagina. Some women may have several consecutive orgasms before experiencing relaxation and pleasure, and some may be unable to reach orgasm at all.

Dyspareunia is genital pain that occurs during or after intercourse when there is not enough lubrication. *Vaginismus* is the involuntary contraction of the vaginal muscles that interferes with vaginal penetration by the penis or fingers.

The most common problem that women report is low sexual desire—30–50% of women seeing sex or marital therapists complain of desire problems.

What causes sexual dysfunctions?

Sexual dysfunctions can be caused by any disease or medication that interferes with the hormones, brain and nerve involvement, blood circulation, or muscles involved in sexual response. Additionally, pain or disability can interfere. Just as important are psychological factors. Physical and emotional factors can interact to cause problems.

What are the symptoms of sexual problems in women with diabetes?

Some women with type 1 diabetes have difficulty becoming physically aroused. They may have less vaginal thickening and lubrication. Both penile erection and vaginal lubrication depend on the increase of blood flow to the genital area. Along with vaginal dryness, an inadequate accumulation of blood in the genital area can cause irritation or pain with sexual activity. Many of these women report using lubricants. Women with type 2 are even more likely to have these problems. Even though their frequency of intercourse and masturbation is the same as women without diabetes, women with type 2 have reported being much less satisfied with almost every aspect of their sexual relationship. Fear of rejection or the negative consequences of future complications affect many women.

What puts you at risk for developing sexual problems?

The damage that high levels of blood glucose in diabetes can do to your blood vessels and nerves affects both circulation and sensation. Clearly, this damage may affect what you can feel and how you respond.

Persistent high blood glucose levels can increase your chance of vaginitis (inflammation of the vagina) or yeast infections. If you have problems with unusual discharge from the vagina, itching, or yeast infections, consult with your doctor to determine the best treatment for correcting the problem and improving your blood glucose control. High blood glucose can also sap your energy and sense of vitality. Feeling sluggish and tired can interfere with how attracted and receptive you are to engaging in sexual activity.

Being able to enjoy the wide range of physical and emotional feelings associated with sexual contact is linked to your emotional state. This can have as powerful an effect on sexual dysfunction as a physical problem.

Women who have multiple health problems may be taking medications that interfere with their ability to have fulfilling sexual contact. Some medications can interfere with your desire to have sex (libido). Others cause drying of the vaginal tissue, which leads to painful intercourse. Ask your doctor about the effects of your medications on your sexual health.

Should you be concerned about diabetes during sex?

If you take insulin or certain diabetes pills (sulfonylureas or meglitinides), the physical exertion of sex might result in low blood glucose. You could reduce the dose of insulin before having sex, or eat something beforehand. If blood glucose goes low, you may find that you are unable to perform as usual and cannot enjoy the experience. Discuss with your partner the potential for low blood glucose, the symptoms, and the treatment, and how to help you.

Does diabetes affect your monthly cycles?

You may have noticed your blood glucose levels are higher around or during your period. Blood glucose is affected by the natural release of hormones that cause your body to be more resistant to its own insulin or to insulin that you inject. Normally, blood glucose remains high for 3–5 days and gradually returns to the level it was before your period.

During PMS, menstruation, and menopause, you might have less energy and not want to exercise. If you stop exercising, your blood glucose may rise even higher. Your ability to control food cravings and to continue with your exercise program will help you balance your blood glucose (and your emotions). Chart your responses during your cycle. Also note the effect of caffeine and alcohol on blood glucose levels at these times. Women with uncontrolled blood glucose may have irregular monthly cycles and acne.

What do your provider and diabetes educator need to know?

Women, especially older ones, are often reluctant to raise the subject of sexual health, believing that their concerns are embarrassing, trivial, or inappropriate unless the provider brings up the topic. It may not be easy to communicate your concerns to your partner or to your provider. Yet, if you want to honor yourself as a woman and this is an issue for you, take the risk. Let your provider know if you have noticed any changes in your sex life. Do you have

- a decrease in sexual desire or interest?
- vaginal dryness or tightness with intercourse?
- pain or discomfort with intercourse?
- soreness and irritation after sexual activity?
- more difficulty reaching an orgasm than in the past?
- less satisfaction with your sexual relationship now than you had before?

To assess the possible emotional causes of your sexual dysfunction, your provider needs to know the following:
1. What was your level of sexual activity and responsiveness (how often, how varied, who initiates it) before diabetes?
2. What are the sexual needs and expectations of you and your partner?
3. What other or underlying difficulties are the two of you having?
4. How do you feel about having diabetes? To what extent does it interfere with your life and relationship?

5. What effect do you feel diabetes has had on your relationship in general and your sexual relationship in particular?

Why is it helpful to know when the problem began?

It helps to know when the sexual problem began to determine what may be the cause and whether it is related to diabetes complications or psychosocial adjustment. It is also helpful to know whether the problem is generalized (occurs in every sexual situation or with different partners) or situational (occurs only during specific sexual activities).

Does your spouse or partner need to speak with your provider?

Of course. Your spouse or sexual partner plays the other important role in the situation. Your partner's viewpoint on any sexual problems or any changes in your sexual relationship might help you find and treat the cause—and improve communication between you. Chronic illness can place stress and strain even on strong relationships. It is important to assess how your partner is affected by the illness, because this can impact your sexual relationship, too.

What can you expect from treatment?

If your sexual problem is mild, began recently, or has a strong diabetes-related cause, some practical and brief interventions by your health care team may be effective.

If your sexual problems are long standing or complicated, you probably need to work with both your physician for treatment of your diabetes and a counselor or therapist in sexual, marital, or individual counseling. You may need accurate sexual education about normal sexual behaviors—there are many excellent books on the subject. It helps many women to realize that their concerns, thoughts, fantasies, and experiences are normal and shared by many other women.

What part do hormones play in the treatment of sexual dysfunction?

A woman who has lost ovarian function or has gone through menopause may experience less desire for sex because of a hormonal deficiency. Estrogen replacement can improve vaginal elasticity and lubrication, but additional supplementation with male sex hormones (androgens) is more likely to directly increase sexual desire. Although androgen therapy has been helpful to women who undergo surgical menopause, it has no documented benefit for premenopausal women with low sexual desire.

The arousal-phase problem of poor vaginal lubrication is often easy to treat. A woman who has low estrogen levels can use replacement estrogen as a pill, patch, or vaginal cream. The estrogen can actually reverse vaginal atrophy within a few months. For premenopausal diabetic women or for those postmenopausal patients who don't take estrogen, vaginal lubricants are quite helpful.

Are there any exercises that help with sexual difficulties?

To minimize pain during intercourse, you can learn to relax the pubococcygeal muscles. You can identify these muscles by contracting them during urination and noticing that the flow stops. You can put a finger inside of the vagina before squeezing the muscles and feel the slight vaginal contraction. Once you have found the muscles, you can practice squeezing them for a count of 3 and then releasing them, 10 times in a row. If vaginal penetration for intercourse feels tight and painful, you can tense and relax the muscles before and during the process. Patients who have pain on penetration or with deep thrusting should use positions that give you more control. These include sitting or kneeling over your partner or both partners lying on your sides facing each other.

Is difficulty in reaching orgasm a separate problem in women with diabetes?

No. Rather, it is often a product of lessened desire and arousal or physical discomfort during sex. Before assuming the trouble is related to neuropathy, your physician may ask if you are orgasmic with clitoral stimulation (by your hand, with a vibrator, or from a partner). Many healthy women have a difficult time reaching orgasm from penile-vaginal thrusting alone, and the woman with orgasmic difficulty may simply require more adequate clitoral stimulation to reach orgasm.

When might you be referred to a specialist?

A referral to a specialist in sexual problems is indicated when:

- The sexual problem is severe or has been present for several years.
- The problem does not respond to primary care provider's treatment.
- The patient is poorly adjusted psychologically or has a highly conflicted close relationship.
- The problem does not appear to be related to diabetes.

For most women's sexual problems, the referral of choice is to a mental health professional who has special training in treating sexual dysfunctions. The most common causes of sexual problems in women with diabetes are psychological—depression, anxiety about attractiveness, poor sexual communication, relationship conflict, or a history of a traumatic sexual experience. The specialist is likely to be a qualified social worker, psychiatrist, or psychologist who has specialty training at the postgraduate level. These professionals can be located on the faculty of a local psychology department or medical school. County or state mental health organizations can also provide referrals. Professional organizations, such as the Society for Sex Therapy and Research, are also sources of reliable referrals.

Can depression cause sexual difficulties?

Loss of desire for sex is often related to depression. If you also have disturbed sleep, a change in appetite for food, depressed mood, chronic fatigue, physical symptoms without clear cause, and trouble with concentration or memory, you probably could benefit from treatment for depression. Antidepressant drugs and brief symptom-focused psychotherapy are both effective. Also, any problem with the couple that decreases communication or increases anger may negatively impact on sexual desire.

When might you be referred to a gynecologist?

A gynecologist is especially helpful with dysfunctions related to menopause or to genital pain. The examination should assess tenderness around the vagina, the condition of Bartholin's glands (which secrete vaginal lubrication), the mucous membranes of the vagina, and the presence of pain deep in the vagina or pelvis with pressure or movement of the cervix and uterus. Women who have vulvar (external genitalia) tenderness, burning, and pain with sexual stimulation sometimes have a syndrome known as *vulvar vestibulitis*. Inflammation of numerous glands around the vaginal opening can be diagnosed with colposcopy. Common causes of pain only on deep thrusting include endometriosis, pelvic adhesions, abnormalities of the uterine ligaments, or ovarian cysts. Only ovarian cysts have been associated with diabetes.

The overproduction of insulin in the insulin resistant state of pre-diabetes or undetected type 2 affects the ovaries and causes polycystic ovarian disease (PCOD), which is usually diagnosed before type 2 diabetes.

Does diabetes affect your choice of contraception?

Options range from abstinence to the pill. In the past, a woman with diabetes was advised against taking the pill for two reasons. First, taking oral contraceptives could worsen her blood glucose control. Even today, a woman may find that this is true. Second, she may be at risk of developing problems with circulation and clotting, such as heart attack or stroke. Because the dose of estrogen and progestin has been decreased in newer pills, so has the risk for these problems. A newly developed progestin counteracts androgen (the male hormone that produces acne in women) and prevents it from stimulating hair growth and oiliness. This progestin is not associated with premenstrual symptoms either—a real plus.

Women on the pill who smoke are at greater risk for circulation problems. Smoking causes the blood vessels to narrow, the walls of the vessels to thicken, and the blood to clot. That's why it is important for a woman to quit smoking. High A1C levels (indicating poor blood glucose control) or being dehydrated may also increase your chances of having blood clotting problems.

A new class of pills for type 2 diabetes, the 'glitazones, can decrease the effectiveness of estrogen by 30%. If you take rosiglitazone or pioglitazone while you are on a low-dose birth control pill, you may have breakthrough bleeding (bleeding between periods) or may even become pregnant. If you are on the pill and taking these drugs, ask your physician if your birth control pill needs to be changed. Also, use a backup method of birth control the first couple of months that you are taking a 'glitazone.

It is important for a woman on the pill to have her blood fats and blood pressure checked regularly. If you have high blood pressure or high blood fats, you may need to use a different method of contraception. Taking the pill when you have high blood pressure can increase the chance that eye or kidney disease will get worse. The pill can also cause a rise in blood cholesterol, LDL, and triglyceride levels. Barrier methods, such as the diaphragm or condoms, have no effect on blood glucose or blood fats. Speak with your provider about the best options for you.

How does diabetes affect pregnancy?

Women with diabetes need to establish near-normal blood glucose levels **before** getting pregnant. The baby's organs (heart, brain, lungs, kidneys, etc.) are formed in the first 8 weeks of pregnancy, often before you know you are pregnant. Good blood glucose control helps protect your baby from birth defects, and keeps you healthy during pregnancy, too. If you maintain normal blood glucose and see your health care team regularly, you and the child should be fine. If you already have complications, especially retinopathy, CAD, or nephropathy, they may get worse, and you and your baby are at higher risk of problems. With your spouse and doctor, weigh the risks before you get pregnant.

You cannot take diabetes pills during pregnancy, so you'll switch to insulin. Taking 3 or more insulin injections a day or using an insulin pump provides you the best chance for normal blood glucose levels. You may need to check your blood glucose more often (6 to 10 times a day). Other medications used in diabetes such as cholesterol-lowering drugs and ACE-inhibitors are also not recommended during pregnancy.

During pregnancy you have an increased risk of headaches, DKA, urinary infections, and preeclampsia.

As soon as you deliver the baby, your insulin needs return to your normal level or you can return to your diabetes pill. If you breastfeed, you may have low blood sugars that are more severe and occur more often than before you were pregnant. See a dietitian before and during pregnancy to be sure you're getting the calories you need. Snacking is important to cover bedtime and middle-of-the-night feedings.

How might your diabetes affect your baby?

If you have near-normal blood glucose levels throughout pregnancy, from conception through delivery, your child has the same low risk of birth defects as any other child. The infant of a mother with diabetes usually weighs more than normal, which can lead to birth injuries, such as a broken collarbone. The baby may have jaundice after birth because his liver is not mature. If your blood glucose is high during labor, she may have hypoglycemia once the cord is cut. This may occur 1–3 hours after birth and should be checked for the first two days of life. Some babies may have breathing difficulties and need oxygen at birth because their lungs have not matured as quickly as they have grown. If you have type 1 diabetes, your child is a little more likely to develop diabetes (1–4%). If you have type 2, your child's risk is 1 in 7. Your child is more likely to be obese after puberty, so give him or her a healthy lifestyle of well-balanced meals and plenty of exercise.

How can pregnancy cause a woman to get diabetes?

Babies in the womb need a different mix of oxygen, sugar, fats, and proteins than their mothers, so hormones are released in the mother's body to get the right mix to the baby. However, these pregnancy hormones make the mother's body resistant to insulin, which causes high blood glucose. The mother's pancreas produces more insulin, but sometimes she can't make enough and her blood levels of glucose, fats, and protein increase. The baby's pancreas reacts to high glucose mixture by producing more insulin, which causes the baby to grow faster than it should.

Women who develop diabetes only during pregnancy, called *gestational diabetes*, do not have the same risks as a woman with diabetes before she gets pregnant. You don't have complications of diabetes, and your baby's organs are formed before the diabetes develops. To keep the baby from being too large, you should follow a meal plan, and you may need insulin to keep your blood glucose normal. Big babies are harder to deliver and you may need a cesarean section (C-section). Your blood glucose should return to normal soon after the birth, but you are more likely to develop type 2 diabetes later on in life.

How are menopause and diabetes connected?

Each woman experiences menopause differently. Your experience will be influenced by your body, your attitudes and fears about menopause, and the thoughts and beliefs of your friends. It is a natural process, but it is a time of unpredictable swings in hormones and emotions. Swings in hormones can cause difficulty sleeping, mood swings, and foggy thinking and can affect your blood glucose control.

The symptoms experienced during menopause can often be confused with the symptoms of low and even high blood glucose. Hot flashes, moodiness, and short-term memory loss can be mistaken as low blood glucose, when in fact they are related to shifts in hormone levels. It is important for you to check your blood glucose level before assuming that it is low and eating unnecessary calories

During menopause, women often report low blood glucose levels that are stronger and more frequent, especially during the middle of the night. Sleep is often disrupted. Controlling your diabetes can be difficult—as it is for teenagers, who also experience wide swings in hormone levels. When the hormone levels increase, blood glucose increases as well. Dealing with the unpredictability of blood glucose and hot flashes can leave you feeling frustrated and sad.

Keep your diabetes regimen going, get adequate sleep and exercise, and try relaxation techniques to help balance the effects of emotional and physical stress. Nap when you need to, and learn to breathe deeply. You might try a yoga class to calm yourself and feel more comfortable in your body. It is important for you to realize that the demands of your diabetes regimen on top of the challenge of hormonal changes and feeling older can change your personality. Try to choose a positive outlook each day and be kind to those around you.

As the levels of the hormones estrogen and progesterone decrease, your body will be less resistant to insulin. Some women experience more hypoglycemia. You may find that you need to decrease the dose of your insulin or diabetes pills during or after menopause. Another body change that you may see during and after menopause is vaginal dryness, resulting in painful intercourse and increased risk for urinary tract infections. Persistent high blood glucose levels can make this condition worse. Cream and gel lubricants can be used during sexual activity. Hormone replacement therapy (HRT) is an option for some women. Prompt treatment of vaginal and urinary tract infections is important. Drink enough water everyday.

Good nutrition, weight training, aerobic exercise, and sleep are the foundation for a healthy transition during menopause. You may want to consider yoga, tai chi, meditation, and other stress reduction techniques to help relieve the symptoms and enhance your overall feeling of well-being.

An RD can help review your needs for calcium supplements and make changes to your meal plan. Some women report that calcium-magnesium supplements help to reduce headaches, irritability, depression, and insomnia. Calcium can be found in high amounts in dairy products; green, leafy vegetables; cauliflower; pinto beans and soybeans; and nuts. The daily requirement for calcium before menopause is 1,000 mg/day. Postmenopausal women need 1,000 mg if they are on HRT and 1,500 mg if they are not. Calcium replacement will also help prevent osteoporosis. Some women report success using a higher soy diet and supplementing with bioflavinoids. If you choose to supplement with herbs, be aware that herbs are like medicines and must be taken under the supervision of someone trained in this area.

How does menopause affect your heart?

Estrogen provides a certain degree of protection against heart disease. Estrogen, released from the ovaries, helps to increase the production of HDL cholesterol, the good cholesterol, and to break down LDL cholesterol, the bad cholesterol. It also relaxes the smooth muscle of the blood vessels. Once a woman experiences menopause, the production of estrogen goes down.

As a woman with diabetes, you are already at risk for developing heart disease earlier. Diabetes negates the protective effects of estrogen and puts you at risk for heart disease and a life-threatening heart attack. If you have heart disease, try to avoid hypoglycemia because of the increased chance of having a heart attack (chapter 5).

Does diabetes put you more at risk for osteoporosis?

As a woman ages, her bones tend to become weaker, putting her at risk for osteoporosis. Yet there are things you can do today to protect your bones.

Osteoporosis, which means "porous bone," is a condition in which bone mass is lost as a result of losing minerals and protein. Bones become very fragile and fracture easily. Estrogen, calcium, vitamin D, and weight-bearing exercise are important to the health and strength of your bones. Even though all humans lose a little bone mass, not all women are at risk for osteoporosis. Men can develop it, too.

You are more at risk for osteoporosis if you are a smoker, thin, fair skinned, have experienced menopause early, have been on steroid therapy, or have had prolonged high blood glucose levels. In addition, if you do not take in enough calories or calcium, or you have a history of anorexia or bulimia, your bones have not received the nutrients they need to stay strong. If you have been caught up in quick-weight-loss diet fads or have a diet low in calcium, high in alcohol and caffeine, or very low in fat, your bones have probably been weakened. Your body needs a little bit of dietary fat to make estrogen, which is needed for building bone and preventing bone loss.

Because most women with type 2 diabetes are overweight, they are less likely to develop osteoporosis. However, this is not true if their blood glucose levels are always high.

How is osteoporosis prevented and treated?

No matter what age you are, you should consider the suggestions below.

- Engage in weight-bearing exercise, which is the best way to increase muscle mass and protect your bones. Your body will respond nicely to exercise that involves repetition and muscle strengthening of the large muscle groups. Even lifting 1 or 2 pounds helps increase bone mass and muscle strength.
- Stop smoking! Smoking interferes with calcium absorption and leaves the bone fragile and thin. Smoking is also a risk because smokers tend to eat a high-fat diet, drink excess alcohol, and exercise less— all risk factors for developing osteoporosis.
- Eat a balanced meal plan that has enough calcium, phosphorus, and vitamin D. Ask a dietitian how you can increase these minerals in your diet.
- Get your diabetes under control!

- Consider HRT or other medications (Calcitonin, Fosamax), especially if you are at high risk or if you are postmenopausal. Explore this option and its side effects with your provider.

Lois Jovanovic, MD; Edward R. Newton, MD; Laurinda M. Poirier, RN, MPH, CDE; Mark A. Sperling, MD; Leslie R. Schover, PhD; Ilana P. Spector, PhD; and Patricia Schreiner-Engel, PhD, contributed to this chapter.

19

Oral Health

Case study

PJ is a 19-year-old woman with type 1 diabetes. She has an abscessed (infected) wisdom tooth, and her dentist has recommended the removal of all four wisdom teeth. The oral surgeon, conferring with PJ's physician, may recommend a temporary reduction in insulin dosage after the extractions, because she won't be able to eat after the surgery. She will be closely monitored to prevent the development of DKA (chapter 1) or hypoglycemia (chapter 2).

Introduction

People with diabetes may develop a variety of oral problems, including gum disease and infections. Seemingly routine dental problems like gum infections and abscesses from bad teeth can have a significant impact on blood sugar levels.

Toothaches, gum disease, or any oral condition that can interfere with your ability to eat takes on added significance. Because healthy eating is such a key element to your control of the disease, it is even more important to maintain a healthy mouth. The key to good oral health is to focus on preventive care through regular checkups and cleanings and an oral hygiene program at home.

How does diabetes affect your mouth and teeth?

Diabetes affects the mouth in three ways:

1. High blood glucose has an effect on the small blood vessels of the body. In the mouth it contributes to gum disease and slower healing.
2. People with diabetes have difficulty fighting off infections in the mouth. Their white blood cells show diminished capacity to fight off invading bacteria.
3. Diabetes can lead to an oral condition known as *xerostomia*, or dry mouth. This decrease in saliva production may be caused by autonomic neuropathy and can have several effects, including more cavities and oral fungal and bacterial infections.

What is periodontal disease?

Periodontal disease may be referred to as *gum disease*, *gingivitis*, or *periodontitis*. These are all terms referring to the breakdown of the structures that support the teeth—the gums and bone.

In a healthy mouth, the roots of the teeth are solidly encased in bone. The soft tissue (the gums) covers the bone and wraps around each tooth up to the base of the crown (Figure 19-1). As a consequence, a space exists around the tooth between it and the gums called the *periodontal pocket*.

Two types of material build up on the teeth above the gumline and below in the pocket: *plaque* and *calculus* (also called tartar). Plaque is a soft film that can be removed with normal brushing and flossing. Calculus is the harder material that is removed by dentists and dental hygienists during regular cleaning sessions. Both are rich in bacteria and cause irritation to the gums. If plaque and calculus are allowed to remain in contact with the teeth and gums, periodontal disease can develop and progress through several stages.

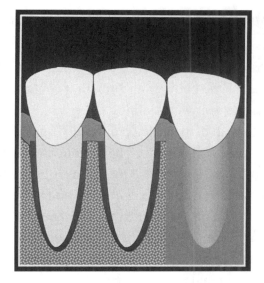

Figure 19-1. Anatomy of healthy teeth/gums/bone. Note the height of the bone and the tightness of the gums against the teeth.
Illustration by Julio Galvez, DDS

What are the symptoms of gum disease?

In gingivitis, the earliest stage of gum disease, the gums are red and swollen and bleed easily. After a thorough cleaning, the gums will return to normal. If the teeth are not cleaned, the gumline will begin to recede, exposing some of the root surface (Figure 19-2). As the gumline continues to move, the level of the bone starts to recede as well. Eventually, the teeth will loosen and need to be extracted or may come out on their own (Figure 19-3). At any point in this progression, a thorough cleaning and the implementation of good oral home care will stop the gum recession and bone loss. However, the lost gum and underlying bone cannot be replaced.

What is the connection between periodontal disease and diabetes?

According to data from the National Health and Nutrition Examination Survey, Americans with diabetes are more than twice as likely as the general population to experience some

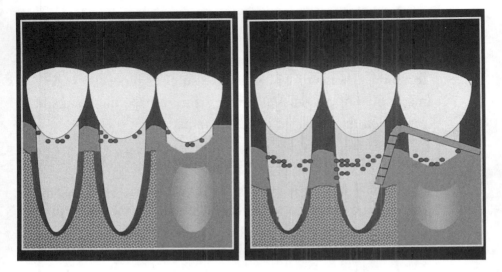

Figures 19-2 and 19-3. Moderate and advanced gum disease. Note the tartar build up and the destruction of bone. We would expect the teeth in figure 19-3 to be loose.
Illustration by Julio Galvez, DDS

form of gum disease. Gum infections can, in turn, significantly raise your blood glucose levels.

How is gum disease diagnosed?

A thorough dental examination includes a visual exam, X rays, and periodontal charting—a series of measurements including the depth of the pocket that surrounds each tooth (Figure 19-3).

What is the treatment for gum disease?

Treatment for gum disease can be as simple as routine cleanings performed every 3–6 months. If the amounts of plaque and calculus are more significant and/or the periodontal pockets are deeper, your dentist may recommend a scaling and root planing. This deep cleaning usually involves several visits and requires a local anesthetic. When completed, you may need to return more frequently than every 6 months for check ups.

In more severe cases, the loss of bony support for the teeth is more extensive, and the depth of the periodontal pockets makes it difficult or impossible to perform a thorough cleaning. You may be referred to a dental specialist concerned with gum problems—the periodontist. The periodontist uses many techniques, some of which involve surgical procedures. A major goal of periodontal surgery is to reshape the bone and reposition the gums for easier cleaning.

How can you prevent gum disease?

Periodontal disease is completely preventable. If plaque and calculus are not allowed to accumulate in the mouth, your gums stay healthy. It is as simple as that.

For most people, this is just a matter of brushing after meals and flossing daily. Electric toothbrushes may be helpful for people who have trouble with regular brushing and flossing. There are prescription products such as medicated rinses and toothpastes designed to kill bacteria and control bleeding and inflammation.

How does dry mouth affect your oral health?

Xerostomia, or dry mouth, is thought to be due to autonomic neuropathy. While a lack of saliva is an annoyance in itself, it can also make you more likely to get cavities in your teeth.

How is dry mouth treated?

Your dentist may prescribe fluoride gels or rinses to strengthen the teeth and fill in small cavities. These products have more fluoride than over-the-counter toothpastes and should only be used with the advice of a dentist. Another prescription product is artificial saliva that can be sipped and swished to aid you in eating and speaking.

Nonprescription techniques include gum, candy, cantaloupe juice, or water. Gum and candies stimulate the flow of saliva. Chewing sugarless gum after meals decreases cavities. Drink more water throughout the day.

Will diabetes interfere with dental treatment?

People with well-controlled diabetes can undergo dental treatment the same as anyone else, although some general precautions should always be taken. Local anesthetic with epinephrine should be avoided on many people with diabetes, especially those who have had diabetes for a long time, because it causes a rapid heartbeat (tachycardia). Ask your dentist about this.

People who take insulin or oral medications are best scheduled for midmorning appointments, after taking their medication and eating a normal breakfast. Check your BG. Always ask how long the numbness will last—your dentist can use shorter-acting anesthetics so you don't have to skip a meal.

People with uncontrolled blood glucose pose a challenge, because of frequent fluctuations in blood glucose levels. Your dentist and physician should consult even for routine dental treatment. If you have heart valve disease, you may need protective doses of antibiotics. Always report any heart problems to your dentist.

What happens after your dental treatment?

Find out how long you can expect to be numb and whether there will be any discomfort as the numbness wears off. These two factors affect your ability to eat and so affect blood glucose. You may need to switch to a soft or liquid diet temporarily, or in extreme cases, the dosage of your medication may need to be reduced. Consult with your physician before you do this. For some patients with diabetes, healing time may be longer. Your dentist may ask to see you for a follow-up visit or may prescribe an antibiotic.

This chapter was written by Jeffrey A. Levin, DMD.

20

Prevention

Case study

DS and HA are Pima Indians. They are cousins. DS lives in the U.S. and works for a construction company. Like most of his neighbors, DS eats a lot of high-fat and sugary foods. He has a sedentary lifestyle when he's not at work. At work, he sits at a desk all day. DS has had type 2 diabetes for 5 years.

HA lives in Mexico, where he and his family farm for a living. Like his neighbors, HA eats a lot of foods high in healthy carbohydrates, such as beans and corn tortillas. Farming keeps him constantly active. HA has normal blood glucose levels.

Case study

At age 42, Kay developed type 2 diabetes. She met with a dietitian, attended education classes at her hospital, scoured the internet for information, and started changing her lifestyle. A year later, she has lost 10 pounds and has an exercise routine she loves. Her doctor congratulates her on successfully controlling her diabetes with diet and exercise. However, she's read about supplements on diabetes web sites and wonders if she should take one to prevent diabetes complications.

Kay talked with her health care provider about dietary supplements. They looked at Kay's food records and found that her diet followed the Food Guide Pyramid in all categories except one: Kay had stopped eating dairy products to lose weight. She really never liked milk, and when she realized that cheese was high in calories and saturated fat, she dropped it too. Kay will start taking a calcium supplement, but she decided to wait for more research on the other supplements.

Introduction

This chapter is about the very real benefits of healthful eating and physical activity. Along with diabetes medications, meal planning and exercise are the keys to preventing or slowing down complications with good blood glucose control. This is important for all people with diabetes.

But meal planning and exercise can also prevent type 2 diabetes from developing at all. Both genetics and environment contribute to the development of type 2 diabetes (Figure 20-1). If one of your parents, siblings, or grandparents has diabetes, you are at increased risk of developing it. Even

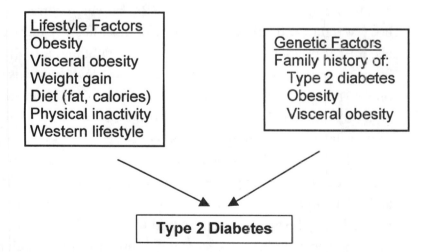

Figure 20-1. Interactions between lifestyle and genetics that can lead to type 2 diabetes.

then, maintaining a healthy body weight and an active lifestyle can help prevent diabetes. A recent study illustrates this point very well. The Pima Indians who live in Arizona have the highest rates of diabetes of any group in the U.S.—75% of the adults have diabetes. They clearly have a strong genetic link to this disease. As the case study shows, the Mexican Pimas have low rates of obesity and low rates of diabetes. Despite a common genetic background, the differences in activity and diet of the two groups create significant differences in how many of them get diabetes.

How do inactivity and obesity increase the risk of diabetes?

Inactivity and obesity make the body less able to use the insulin it produces. It is insulin resistant. For a while, the pancreas overcomes insulin resistance by making more insulin, and blood glucose remains normal. Over time, the pancreas can't keep producing these higher levels of insulin, so blood glucose levels rise, and diabetes develops. Increasing physical activity and a weight loss of even 10 to 20 pounds can improve how the body uses the insulin it does make.

What levels of body weight are associated with diabetes?

Today, we use the body mass index (BMI), which corrects body weight for height (Table 20-1). In most healthy individuals, a BMI of 25–29.9 is considered overweight and a BMI of 30 or more is considered obese. These cutoff levels are based on several large studies. This does not apply to well-trained athletes, who may have a higher BMI because of high levels of muscle mass or to pregnant women.

A BMI above 25 may be too high if you already have medical conditions including type 2 diabetes, high blood pressure, and high cholesterol. People with these health problems or a strong family history of them, should try for a BMI of less than 25. Some studies suggest that the lowest risk of developing diabetes occurs at a BMI of approximately 21.

Table 20.1 Body Mass Index (BMI) Values

BMI

Weight (in pounds)

Height	Good Weights									Increasing Risk													
	19	20	21	22	23	24	25	26	27	28	29	30	31	32	33	34	35	36	37	38	39	40
4'10"	91	96	100	105	110	115	119	124	129	134	138	143	148	153	158	162	167	172	177	181	186	191
4'11"	94	99	104	109	114	119	124	128	133	138	143	148	153	158	163	168	173	178	183	188	193	198
5'	97	102	107	112	118	123	128	133	138	143	148	153	158	163	168	174	179	184	189	194	199	204
5'1"	100	106	111	116	122	127	132	137	143	148	153	158	164	169	174	180	185	190	195	201	206	211
5'2"	104	109	115	120	126	131	136	142	147	153	158	164	169	175	180	186	191	196	202	207	213	218
5'3"	107	113	118	124	130	135	141	146	152	158	163	169	175	180	186	191	197	203	208	214	220	225
5'4"	110	116	122	128	134	140	145	151	157	163	169	174	180	186	192	197	204	209	215	221	227	232
5'5"	114	120	126	132	138	144	150	156	162	168	174	180	186	192	198	204	210	216	222	228	234	240
5'6"	118	124	130	136	142	148	155	161	167	173	179	186	192	198	204	210	216	223	229	235	241	247
5'7"	121	127	134	140	146	153	159	166	172	178	185	191	198	204	211	217	223	230	236	242	249	255
5'8"	125	131	138	144	151	158	164	171	177	184	190	197	203	210	216	223	230	236	243	249	256	262
5'9"	128	135	142	149	155	162	169	176	182	189	196	203	209	216	223	230	236	243	250	257	263	270
5'10"	132	139	146	153	160	167	174	181	188	195	202	209	216	222	229	236	243	250	257	264	271	278
5'11"	136	143	150	157	165	172	179	186	193	200	208	215	222	229	236	243	250	257	265	272	279	286
6'	140	147	154	162	169	177	184	191	199	206	213	221	228	235	242	250	258	265	272	279	287	294
6'1"	144	151	159	166	174	182	189	197	204	212	219	227	235	242	250	257	265	272	280	288	295	302
6'2"	148	155	163	171	179	186	194	202	210	218	225	233	241	249	256	264	272	280	287	295	303	311
6'3"	152	160	168	176	184	192	200	208	216	224	232	240	248	256	264	272	279	287	295	303	311	319
6'4"	156	164	172	180	189	197	205	213	221	230	238	246	254	263	271	279	287	295	304	312	320	328

BMI ≥27 are highlighted because health risk escalates rapidly above this level.

Where body fat is located is also important. An increased amount of fat in the abdomen (apple shape) is more strongly associated with diabetes than is body fat on the hips (pear shape). Abdominal obesity is also associated with high blood pressure, high triglycerides, low levels of HDL "good" cholesterol, and heart disease. In fact, this combination of health problems is serious and is called Syndrome X or Dysmetabolic Syndrome.

Men have more abdominal fat than women. And families often resemble each other in fat patterns. Several behavioral factors increase abdominal obesity, including low physical activity, smoking, stress, and eating a lot of high-fat foods.

To see whether you have abdominal obesity measure your waist. More than 35 inches in women or 40 inches in men suggests that you have abdominal obesity.

Studies have shown that weight gain since age 18 is another important factor in determining the risk of diabetes. People who have gained more than 20 pounds since age 18 are at increased risk of developing diabetes—and it is common for people to gain weight as they age.

How does your diet increase your risk of diabetes?

Eating too much sugar is not the problem. Most studies suggest that it is the amount of fat in the diet, rather than the amount of carbohydrate, that increases the risk of diabetes. Be aware of the amount of fat you are eating for several reasons. First, fat is fattening. Each gram of fat (a gram is about the weight of a paper clip) provides 9 calories. Compare that to the 4 calories in each gram of carbohydrate (fruits, grains, vegetables) and the 4 calories in each gram of protein (meats, fish, poultry). Gram for gram, fat is twice as fattening as carbohydrates or protein. Dietary fats, especially saturated fat, can also raise your cholesterol levels and increase your heart risk.

How do you turn nutrition guidelines into healthy meals?

Guidelines are great, but the real question is, "What should I eat? Which foods will help me control blood sugars and lipid levels, reduce the risk of complications, and promote health and well-being?" A healthy diet is the same for everyone, including people with diabetes. The Food Guide Pyramid illustrates this kind of healthy eating pattern. The ADA has developed a similar pyramid for people with diabetes. The number of servings from each food group depends on the number of calories you require. This is determined by your body size and activity level (Table 20-2). It's best to see a registered dietitian (RD) to develop a meal plan that suits your tastes, your schedule, and your health goals, so you'll know how many servings of each food group to have each day.

You can check your diet to see if you have healthy eating habits. Write down everything you eat for two or three days, then compare each day's log to the Food Guide Pyramid. (The reason for looking at a couple of days is that you may eat less from one group one day, but more the next, so that the average is right on target.) The American Diabetes Association's website, www.diabetes.org, offers tips on changing your eating patterns to match the recommendations of the pyramid. An RD can help you tailor your meal plans to lower blood glucose or lipids, as well as to make adjustments for your food preferences or lifestyle.

What are the healthiest foods to eat?

To get the nutrients you need to eat whole foods, such as vegetables, fruits, and whole grains. Processed foods have lost vitamins and often have had fat, salt, and extra sugar added. In general, avoid white flour, sugar, and salt, and add colors (and vitamins, minerals, and fiber) to your diet with vegetables and fruit.

Table 20-2. Suggested Daily Servings of the Different Food Groups

	Desire weight loss†	Many older women	Women, older adults	Larger women, older men	Children, teen girls, active women, most men	Teen boys, active men
Calorie level	About 1200	About 1400	About 1600	About 1800	About 2200	About 2800
Calorie range	1200–1500	1300–1600	1400–1700	1600–1900	1800–2300	2200–2800
Carbohydrate grams	180	180	195	210	240	300
Carbohydrate choices	12	12	13	14	16	20
Grains, beans, and starchy vegetables	6	6	6	7	9	11
Vegetables	3	3	3	4	4	5
Fruits	3	3	3	3	3	4
Milk‡	2	2	2–3	2–3	2–3	2–3
Meats	2 (4 oz)	2 (4 oz)	2 (5 oz)	2 (5 oz)	2 (6 oz)	3 (7 oz)
Fats g/servings (based on 30% of calories as fat)	40/4	47/5	54/6	60/7	74/9	93/12

* Chart adapted from *Diabetes Meal Planning Made Easy*, 2nd ed. American Diabetes Association. 2000.

† Some older women and men who are small in stature and sedentary may need to eat no more than 1200 calories to lose weight. At 1200 calories, you may need a vitamin and mineral supplement that provides 100% of the Daily Value to meet your nutrition needs.

‡ Teenagers, young adults to age 24, and women who are pregnant or breastfeeding and sedentary may need to eat no more than 1200 calories to lose weight. Adults younger than 50 need 1000 mg of calcium per day. Each cup of milk or yogurt contains about 300 mg of calcium. Other sources of calcium are calcium-fortified orange juice, other dairy products, and dark green leafy vegetables. If you do not get sufficient calcium from the foods you eat, talk to your health care provider about taking a calcium supplement to meet your requirements for calcium. Each serving of milk is equivalent to about 12 grams of carbohydrate or roughly 1 carbohydrate choice.

To develop individualized recommendations about the amount of carbohydrate you should eat at meals and snacks, work with a dietitian or diabetes educator with expertise in diabetes and carbohydrate counting.

If you want to lower blood lipids with dietary changes, see an RD for help. You might try the Mediterranean diet. The emphasis is on fresh foods and olive oil, a monounsaturated (heart healthy) fat. Fresh fruits and vegetables are combined with small amounts of cheese, fish, or lean meat; small servings of fresh bread or pasta; and a glass of wine with the meal. Or you might just cut the saturated fat in your diet to less than 10% of the calories you eat each day, and try eating healthier fats such as olive oil and nuts. Another step is to cut out processed foods with trans fats in them (hydrogenated oils on the food label) to help protect your heart, too.

Research does not show that limiting protein helps protect you against kidney disease. Do not restrict protein below recommended levels, because your body needs it for growth and repair. If you have kidney disease, see an RD for an individualized meal plan. Fish is a good source of protein because it also has omega-3 fatty acids that are heart friendly fats. Soy foods are also good sources of protein that are heart friendly.

Do vitamin and mineral supplements help with diabetes?

Food is better than supplements. We cannot put into a pill all the important substances that foods have. So, if you eat mostly unprocessed foods in a meal plan that your RD designed for you, chances are that you do not need supplements. If you are taking supplements, please tell your health care provider, because these drugs can have an effect on the action of other medications you may be taking. The supplements that Kay read about and that you may have heard about in connection with diabetes are chromium, vanadyl sulfate (vanadium), magnesium, vitamin E, and niacin (vitamin B-3) and other B vitamins. Except for niacin, the ADA does not recommend that you take any of these supplements.

The research on chromium and diabetes has not shown that it helps people with diabetes get better BG control. If you want to include natural sources of chromium in your diet, try whole grains, cheese, beans, nuts, seeds, mushrooms, beef, wheat germ, and broccoli.

Research studies of vanadium also have given mixed results, so it is not recommended. There are GI side effects because even small doses can be toxic. Natural food sources include black pepper, dill, parsley, mushrooms, spinach, oysters, shellfish, cereals, fish and wine.

Studies of magnesium show that it is connected to diabetes complications, but we don't know how. It is not easy to measure magnesium levels in the body, but it is one of the more common deficiencies seen with both types of diabetes. Factors that would increase your risk of being deficient in magnesium are DKA, medications such as diuretics, gastroparesis, renal insufficiency, CHF, heart attack, acute critical illness, alcohol abuse, and pregnancy. People eating low calorie and poor quality diets are more likely to be low in magnesium. Do not take magnesium supplements, not even antacids or laxatives, if you have impaired kidney function. Foods that contain magnesium are whole grains, leafy green vegetables, legumes, nuts, and fish. An unhealthy diet high in saturated fat, fructose, caffeine, and alcohol may increase a person's magnesium needs.

Vitamin E is another supplement that yields mixed results in studies. It may help prevent heart disease—or it may not. It does have anticoagulant properties, so if you are taking medications or supplements that decrease blood clotting, such as warfarin, aspirin, gingko biloba, garlic, and ginseng, you may be at increased risk for bleeding with high-dose supplements. Good food sources of vitamin E are higher-fat foods, such as vegetable oils, margarine, wheat germ, seeds, and nuts. If you are taking a medication such as orlistat, which decreases fat absorption, you may need a vitamin E supplement.

Niacin (vitamin B-3) comes in two forms: nicotinic acid and nicotinamide. It is effective at lowering cholesterol, but it can raise BG levels. The European Nicotinamide Diabetes Intervention Trial (ENDIT) is studying whether niacin preserves beta cell function and prevents or slows the development of type 1 and type 2 diabetes. The study will not be completed until 2003. Niacin causes flushing of the face right after it is taken and may aggravate gallbladder disease, gout, and allergies. Try foods containing niacin such as fortified grains, cereals, meats, fish, and beans.

Another B vitamin mentioned in connection with diabetes is folate or folic acid. Your risk for being deficient in this vitamin is increased by pregnancy and lactation, alcoholism, anorexia, older age, chronic use of certain medications, and gastrointestinal surgery. Folate is widely available in foods but as much as 50–95% of it may be destroyed by processing. Do not take supplements without your doctor's advice, as it may hide a vitamin B-12 deficiency. For best health, eat foods containing B vitamins and reduce alcohol intake and smoking. All "enriched" grain products such as breads, cereals, and pasta, contain folate. Other sources of folate are spinach, orange juice, strawberries, and peanuts. Sources of B-12 are animal products, and good sources of B-6 include whole grains, animal products, and legumes.

How does physical activity affect diabetes?

In the Nurses Health Study, more than 80,000 nurses aged 35–59 were followed for 8 years. Women who engaged in vigorous activity at least one time per week had a lower risk of developing diabetes than those who were less active. In fact, the major difference was between the women who reported no physical activity and those who exercised at least one time per week.

Being inactive increases the chance that you will be overweight, and being overweight increases your risk of diabetes.

However, even if you adjust for this (looking at a group of people all of the same weight), you will find that those people who are most active have the lowest risk of diabetes. This is probably because physical activity makes your body more sensitive to insulin (reduces insulin resistance), and decreases the chance that you will develop type 2 diabetes. Exercise also helps reduce abdominal obesity, another risk factor for diabetes.

Exercise is the magic "pill" that everyone wants. Participation in regular physical activity offers many health benefits when you have diabetes. It

- lowers blood glucose levels after exercise
- helps the body use insulin better
- makes your heart healthier
- lowers triglyceride levels
- raises HDL, or "good" cholesterol levels
- lowers blood pressure
- helps you lose weight and keep it off
- reduces stress and anxiety
- improves mood

Why is weight loss recommended?

We now know that weight loss of just 10–20 pounds can improve blood glucose, blood pressure, and cholesterol in patients with type 2 diabetes and reduce the risks of heart disease. The benefits of weight loss on blood sugar control occur very quickly and dramatically. Just one or two weeks of eating fewer calories can markedly lower BG levels. If you are using insulin or diabetes pills, notify your physician before starting on a weight-loss program. He or she may want to adjust the dose of insulin or diabetes pills that you are taking and your hypertension medication before the start of the weight-loss program and as you lose weight.

The only way to maintain the positive benefits of weight loss is to maintain your new body weight. This means

continuing to eat a healthy diet and to exercise. If you lose
10–20 pounds and keep it off, you improve your blood glucose, blood pressure, and lipids long term.

What is the treatment for obesity?

The primary treatment for obesity is lifestyle change, involving both food choices and physical activity. Many people find it helpful to have the support of a group in making these changes (for example, TOPS, Weight Watchers, Overeaters Anonymous, or your diabetes support group).

The following suggestions may be helpful:

1. To lose weight, you need to change the energy balance—the amount of energy (calories) you eat and the amount of energy you use up through exercise. The most effective approach to long-term weight loss is to change both sides of the energy-balance equation: eat less and exercise more.

2. To get an idea of what you are currently eating, write down everything you eat for 1 week. Be careful to write down *everything,* and be precise about describing the food and the serving size. Use a calorie and fat guide or the food label to figure out how many calories and grams of fat you are eating.

3. To lose weight, you need to eat less than you are currently eating. To lose 1–2 pounds per week, which is considered the best rate of weight loss, you need to reduce the amount of calories you are eating by 500–1,000 calories per day. If you find that you usually eat 2,000 calories, you should eat 1,000–1,500 calories/day to lose weight. Do not go below 1,100 calories per day because it is hard to eat a healthy diet below this level. To get as much food as possible at a calorie level, consider eating less fat so you can have more of other foods. See an RD to develop a balanced meal plan for you.

4. Increase your physical activity in the form of brisk walking. Check with your physician before beginning any physical activity more vigorous than walking. Start slowly and build up gradually to avoid injury. *Any* physical activity burns calories. You don't need to jog a mile to burn calories; walking the mile works just as well. You can take three short walks of 10 minutes each. Gradually increase your activity until you are walking for a total of 30 minutes each day.

5. Set up your home to support your healthier lifestyle. It is easier to follow an eating plan if you buy healthy foods and have them available. Don't purchase high-fat snack items such as chips, crackers, nuts, or cheese. The principle is: "Out of sight is out of mind." Do the reverse for physical activity. If you own an exercise bike, put it where you'll use it. Keep your walking shoes by the door.

6. Set a goal of losing 10–20 pounds and keeping it off. Losing 10–20 pounds reduces the risk of obesity-related health problems and helps treat those problems.

Are there medications for the treatment of obesity?

Several medications promote weight loss by helping you eat less or by blocking the absorption of the fat you eat. However, for them to work, they must be used with changes in diet and physical activity.

Weight losses with prescription medication have averaged 5–15 pounds higher than those seen with nondrug treatments, but the maximum weight loss typically occurs at 6 months, followed by a plateau in weight or regaining the weight.

Weight loss medications are recommended primarily for people who are significantly obese or have health problems associated with their obesity. These medications, like all medications, have side effects. Most of the side effects are mild, but you should consult your physician before using any of them. Don't use them if you want to lose just a few pounds.

How can you learn more about weight and physical activity?

There is a tremendous amount of misinformation available about obesity and physical activity. Useful and accurate information can be obtained from the Weight-Control Information Network (WIN). WIN is a service of the National Institute of Diabetes and Digestive and Kidney Diseases, a division of the National Institutes of Health. They can be contacted at:

Weight-Control Information Network
1 Win Way, Bethesda, MD 20892-3665
Phone: (800) 946-8098
Fax: (301) 570-2186

Does diabetes put you at risk for eating disorders?

Although some people with diabetes do develop full-fledged eating disorders—anorexia nervosa, bulimia, and binge-purging—more common are eating disturbances. Symptoms of eating disturbances include:

- drastically reducing your calorie intake
- cutting back on or skipping your insulin
- skipping diabetes pills as a weight-control measure
- thinking about food all the time
- a strong fear of gaining weight
- bingeing
- using laxatives or vomiting on purpose to control weight
- exercising excessively

Unfortunately, eating disturbances make you less healthy. Insulin underdosing is dangerous because it causes high BG levels and can easily lead to DKA. Likewise, skipping diabetes pills lets BG levels run high and increases your risk of complications. If you think that you have an eating disturbance, take action. A therapist can help you revamp your thoughts and attitudes and enjoy a healthier relationship with your food.

What safety measures should you take for exercising with complications such as neuropathy?

Your best exercise options are non-weight-bearing activities such as swimming, bicycling, rowing, armchair exercises (stretching, light weightlifting, and sitting aerobics), t'ai chi, yoga, stretching, and moderate strengthening with exercise bands or balls.

Avoid these activities: Weight-bearing activities, especially those that are high impact, strenuous, or prolonged, such as walking a distance, jogging or running, treadmill exercise, high impact aerobics, stair climbing, jumping or hopping, starting and stopping, and side-to-side type activities (like singles tennis or basketball).

Protect your feet: do visual checks of your feet before and after exercising, and wear well-fitting footwear.

What should you watch for with autonomic neuropathy?

When autonomic neuropathy affects the heart and cardiovascular system, the way your blood pressure and heart rate respond to changes in activity may be affected. It may take longer than usual at the start of an exercise session for your heart rate and blood pressure to increase. You may have less tolerance for intense exercise, and your heart rate and blood pressure at the end of an exercise session may be unpredictable. Always warm-up before and cool-down after exercising, exercise at a moderate intensity, avoid rapid posture changes that can cause lightheadedness and dizziness, and don't do heavy lifting or straining.

Exercise that is too vigorous or "hard" is especially risky when you have autonomic neuropathy. Make certain that you can carry on a conversation while you exercise! Supervised exercise may be your safest option. Always talk with your physician and have a cardiovascular evaluation before starting a new exercise routine.

If neuropathy has affected your sweating mechanisms and body temperature regulation, you can get overheated or even develop heat stroke. Pay careful attention to the weather and drink enough fluids. Make an effort to drink 1/2 cup of fluid about every 15 minutes during exercise and avoid exercising in extreme temperatures and high humidity.

What are your exercise options with retinopathy?

Your best exercise options are moderate activity including stationary cycling, swimming, walking, low-intensity machine rowing. Avoid strenuous activities like jogging, running, and high-impact aerobics or ones that involve vigorous bouncing or jarring; contact sports; heavy weightlifting with high resistance and low repetitions; isometric exercise; holding your breath during exertion; strenuous upper body and arm exercise; or any activities that lower your head below your waist.

Very strenuous exercise of any kind can cause excessive increases in blood pressure. This, in turn, can increase the pressure in the eye and can cause hemorrhaging, especially in eyes that are already damaged. Keep your head UP!

Is it safe to exercise if you have nephropathy?

Though exercise is in many ways beneficial, it does cause a short-term increase in blood pressure, which in turn leads to changes in renal function, including an exercise-related increase in protein excretion in the urine. Though these changes are short-lived, just what they mean in terms of the progression of kidney disease is still being debated. We do know that protein in the urine as a result of exercise can be reduced when blood glucose control is at its best and when blood pressure is also under control.

If you have advanced nephropathy, your ability to exercise may be limited because of anemia, muscle weakness, and changes in how your heart responds to exercise. Even so, doing mild or moderate activity can help improve your ability to function independently, improve your mood, and reduce feelings of anxiety and depression.

The best exercise options with nephropathy are light or moderate daily activity, such as light household chores, gardening, walking, water exercise, stretching, easy calisthenics, or light weightlifting. This is because when you exercise, the amount that blood pressure increases is related to how difficult the session is or how long it lasts (the more taxing the activity, the more blood pressure will go up).

What exercises keep your heart healthy?

Because diabetes greatly increases your risk of heart and vascular diseases, have a medical examination to assess the health of your heart and circulatory system before you begin a new exercise routine. The exam should include an evaluation of your blood pressure, the circulation in your feet and legs (chapter 10), and a graded exercise, or stress, test (chapter 5) if you:

- are over age 35
- have had type 2 diabetes for more than 10 years
- have had type 1 diabetes for more than 15 years
- have any additional risk factors for coronary artery disease (see Chapter 5), including obesity, high LDL cholesterol, low HDL cholesterol, and smoking
- have microvascular disease (proliferative retinopathy or nephropathy, including microalbuminurea, and peripheral neuropathy)

- have peripheral vascular disease
- have autonomic neuropathy

A stress test shows how your heart and blood pressure respond to exercise. The results can help your doctor identify a safe level of exercise for you, including an appropriate heart-rate range, best types of activities, and special exercise precautions. It should be repeated every 3 years. Abnormal electrocardiogram changes and/or blood pressure responses that occur before, during, or after exercise may indicate the need for special precautions or limitations.

Avoid high-intensity activity, heavy weightlifting with few repetitions, isometric exercise, or lifting while holding your breath. To be safe exercise consistently and regularly rather than erratically, and gradually increase your exercise routine. Monitor your heart rate when you exercise (a range of 60–80% of the maximum heart rate achieved during a stress test is recommended, but your physician should give you your own range). Achieve good blood pressure control before exercising and monitor how your blood pressure responds to activity. When you are just beginning, monitor your blood sugar before, during, and after exercise. Check before and after to be sure your BG is not too high or too low. Avoid exercising in extreme heat, cold or humidity; and consider indoor exercise when the weather is extreme or air quality is poor.

Your best exercise options are moderate-intensity aerobic activity such as walking, cycling, jogging, swimming, lifting light weights with many repetitions (at least 8 to 15 repetitions), and stretching. Walking (or other weight-bearing exercise) is preferred if you have mild to moderate peripheral vascular disease and claudication—exercise until you can't tolerate the discomfort, then stop for a period of rest before resuming exercise. If you can't do weight-bearing activity (as with peripheral neuropathy) there are seated aerobics and stretching programs. Swimming may work for you, too. Supervised exercise in a cardiac rehabilitation program is advisable if you have chest pain with exertion, heart failure, or have had a recent heart attack, angioplasty, or bypass surgery. Supervised exercise is also recommended if you have severe peripheral vascular disease.

Any kind of exercise makes your heart healthier. Do the best you can to find activities that work for you.

This chapter was written by Rena R. Wing, PhD; Katherine V. Williams, MD; Charlotte Hayes, MMSc, MS, RD, CDE; and Joan M. Heins, MA, RD, CDE.

Appendix A:
Regular Checkups

Complication	What to do	Target
A1C	Twice a year	Below 7
Blood pressure	At each visit	Below 130/80
Cholesterol (LDL)	Once a year	Below 100
Eyes	Yearly dilated eye exam	
Kidneys	Yearly microalbumin and clearance test	
Nerves	Yearly check with monofilaments	
Feet	Check for neuropathy and foot deformity at least twice a year	
Heart	Stress test if indicated	
Teeth	Cleaning and check-up twice a year	

Good CENSE

Have good CENSE about your diabetes. The "C" in CENSE stands for Control. That includes blood sugar control, blood pressure control, and cholesterol (lipids) control. For blood sugar an A1C test is done quarterly and you want it as near normal as possible. Blood pressure should be checked at each doctor's office visit, and it should be less than 130/80. Lipids are checked once a year, and you want an LDL (bad) cholesterol level of less than 100, HDL (good) cholesterol of greater than 45, and a triglyceride level of less than 200.

The first "E" in CENSE stands for Early treatment—which, of course, requires that you find the condition early—of eyes, heart, kidneys, and feet. To find problems early get these check-ups: for your eyes, have a yearly dilated eye examination; for your heart, take aspirin and get stress testing when needed; for kidneys, have a yearly microalbumin test; and for your feet, have a yearly check with a monofilament.

The "NS" in CENSE stands for No Smoking. It gets two letters because it is so important.

The last "E" in CENSE stands for Education. Diabetes education, nutrition education, and exercise education are all essential to your good health. Go when you are diagnosed, and brush up on the latest developments every three years.

These are not "Best Care" recommendations but rather minimum standards of care. Your diabetes team wants the very best for you. Don't accept or be satisfied with less.

Index

Blood vessel disease, 86, 109, 117, 147–155, 235, 238, 239
Body mass index (BMI), 272–274
Brain attacks, See stroke.
Bruit, 97, 113–114
Bulimia, 230, 262, 283
Bunion, 25–26
Bypass surgery, 79–81, 154–155

C

CAT SCAN, 100
Calcium, 260, 261
Calcium-channel blockers, 78, 119
Calluses, 25–26
Cancer, 96
Candida, 211–213, 216–217
Cane, 30–31
Capsaicin, 162, 164
Carbohydrate, 20,
Cardiac catheterization, 75
Carotid endarterectomy, 98
Carpal tunnel syndrome, 177–179
Casts, 30
Cataracts, 50, 64
CBC, 114
Certified Diabetes Educator (CDE), 115
Charcot's joint, 27
Cholesterol, 49, 71, 77–78, 80–81, 86, 89–96, 108, 110, 112, 115, 130, 148, 236, 244, 257, 261, 271, 274, 278, 280
Circulation, poor, 23–24, 147, 151, 235
Claudication, 28, 75, 112, 147, 150, 151, 235
Clearance, 131
Coma, 12
Computed tomography (CT)scan, 97
Congestive heart failure (CHF), 278
Constipation, 182, 190–191
Contraception, 256–257
Coping, 222–224
Coronary artery disease (CAD), 70–81, 85, 152, 172
Coronary heart disease (CHD), 90,104, 121

Cortisol, 15
Counseling, 252
Cryotherapy, 56, 58
Cystitis, 199

D

Dental care, 264–269
Depression, 236, 238–239, 254–255, 260
Diabetes, 86, 91, 93, 99–100, 109
Diabetes Control and Complications Trial (DCCT), 158
Diabetes pills, 18–19
Diabetic ketoacidosis (DKA), 1–11, 264, 268
Diabetic macular edema, 49
Dialysis, 137–139
Diarrhea, 181–182, 187–189
Diet, 92, 109, 112, 117, 135, 247, 274–277
Dietitian. See registered dietitian.
Digoxen, 87
Diuretics, 118, 127, 171, 238, 278
Driving, 17, 21
Dye, 14, 51–52, 76, 136

E

Eating disorders, 230–232
Echo Cardiogram, 75, 86
Edema, 114, 133, 150, 170–171
Education, 123, 223–224
Elderly, 13, 124
Electrocardiogram (ECG), 74, 102
Endarterectomy, 153
Epinephrine, 15, 171, 174, 269
Erectile dysfuntion, 234–245
ESRD, 134
Estrogen, 260–261
Exercise, 19–20, 68, 165, 75, 92, 112, 116, 165, 247, 250, 260, 280
Eye diseases, 45–69, 121
Eye Exams, 69

F

Fat, 89–90, 209, 258, 274–277, 281
Feet, 22–44, 284

Magnetic resonance imaging (MRI), 29, 100, 101
Meal planning, 274–278
Medicare, 40, 42–43
Menopause, 250, 253, 259–261
Men, 103
Men's sexual health, 234–245
Metformin (Glucophage), 14, 19
Microalbuminuria, 131
Mononeuropathy, 67, 176

N

Nails, 201
Nausea, 83, 127, 185
Necrobiosis Lipidica Diabeticorum(NUD), 206–207
Nephropathy, 118, 120,127–146, 257
Nephrons, 129
Nephrotic syndrome, 133
Neurogenic bladder, 137
Neuropathy,
    autonomic neuropathy, 158, 166–179, 265
    peripheral neuropathy, 23, 156–165
Nicotinic acid, 95, 278
Nonproliferative retinopathy, 48
Nitrogylcerin, 76
Nursing home personnel, 13
Nuts, 79

O

Obesity, 71, 117, 125, 148, 271, 281–283
Opthalmologist, 45, 50
Optic nerve, 67
Oral agents, 18–19,
Oral health, 264–269
Orthostatic hypotension, 73, 113, 118, 125, 170–172
Orthotics, 40
Osteomylitis, 32
Osteoporosis, 261–262
Over the counter medications, 111, 136, 162
Overweight, 115, 272–274, 279

P

Pancreas transplant, 140–146

Patient education, 34, 223–224, 283
Pedorthist, 40–42
Periodontal disease, 265–268
Peripheral neuropathy, 114, 156–165, 238
Peripheral vascular disease (PVD), 121, 147–155, 205
Physical activity. See Exercise.
Pioglitazones, 19, 256
Podiatrist, 19, 256
Polycystic, 255
Prednisone, 1, 12
Pregnancy, 246–247
Prevention, 270–289
Proliferative retinopathy, 48, 127
Prostate gland, 129
Protein, 246, 258
Proteinuria, 115, 133
Psychosocial complications, 219, 233

R

Registered dietitian (RD), 93, 102, 115, 127
Renovascular hpertension, 111
Retina, 48
Retinopathy, 48–63, 121, 128, 235, 246
Rheumatic fever, 100
Rheumatic heart disease, 85
Rosiglitazones, 19, 256
Rotablator, 80

S

Salt, 275
Saturated fats, 278
Screening tests, 46, 50–51, 74, 91, 100–102
Seeds, 79
Sexual dysfunction, 122, 234–245, 247–249, 250
Shoe inserts, 40
Shoes, 28, 33, 35–43
Skin, 204–218
Smoking, vi, 27, 71, 91–92, 96, 105, 112, 117, 130, 146, 240, 244, 256, 251–262, 274
Snacks, 18, 20–21
Socks, 39

Sphygmomanometer, 123
Statins, 93–95
Stents, 80, 88, 108
Sternum, 81
Steroids, 210
Stress, 239
Stress hormones, 15
Stress test, 74–75, 88, 117,
Stroke, 12, 67, 84, 96–108
Sulfonylurea drugs, 18–19, 156, 175
Sweating, 173–174

T

Teeth, 264–269
Tendral, 155
TENS units, 163, 165
Therapeutic Shock Bill (TSB), 42
Thiazolidinediones, 126
TIA, 98, 108
Tissue plasminogen activator (TPA), 84, 102
Transplants, 140–146
Triglycerides, 91, 96, 115, 257, 274
Type 1, 1, 63, 83, 127, 18, 130, 132, 136, 160, 181, 184, 186, 234, 246
Type 2, 49, 63, 83, 97, 125, 147, 132, 136, 156, 158, 180, 184, 246, 249, 255, 256, 262, 270, 271, 279, 280

U

Ulcers, foot, 22, 28–34, 147, 198
Ultrasound, 52
United Netwrok for Organ Sharing (UNOS), 144

Unsaturated fats,
Uremia, 134, 185, 210
Ureters, 129
Urinary tract infection (UTI), 130, 169, 257. 260
Urine ketone test, 4, 10–11

V

Vaginal dryness, 249
Valsalva maneuver, 73, 172
Vascular disease. See blood vessel disease.
Vascular surgeon, 147
Vegetables, 78–79
Vitamins, 78, 89
Vitrectomy, 56. 59–60
Vitreous hemorrhage, 56
Vomitting, 10, 82. 182, 185, 283

W

Walker, 30–31
Warfarin, 107
Weight loss, 94, 116, 185
Women, 91–92, 103, 125
Women's Sexual Health, 246–263
World Health Organization, 10

X

X-rays, 14, 29, 76, 86, 136, 184, 191, 200, 201

Y

Yeast infections, 211–213

About the American Diabetes Association

The American Diabetes Association is the nation's leading voluntary health organization supporting diabetes research, information, and advocacy. Its mission is to prevent and cure diabetes and to improve the lives of all people affected by diabetes. The American Diabetes Association is the leading publisher of comprehensive diabetes information. Its huge library of practical and authoritative books for people with diabetes covers every aspect of self-care—cooking and nutrition, fitness, weight control, medications, complications, emotional issues, and general self-care.

To order American Diabetes Association books: Call 1-800-232-6733. http://store.diabetes.org [Note: there is no need to use **www** when typing this particular Web address]

To join the American Diabetes Association: Call 1-800-806-7801. www.diabetes.org/membership

For more information about diabetes or ADA programs and services: Call 1-800-342-2383. E-mail: Customerservice@diabetes.org www.diabetes.org

To locate an ADA/NCQA Recognized Provider of quality diabetes care in your area: www.ncqa.org/dprp/

To find an ADA Recognized Education Program in your area: Call 1-888-232-0822. www.diabetes.org/recognition/education.asp

To join the fight to increase funding for diabetes research, end discrimination, and improve insurance coverage: Call 1-800-342-2383. www.diabetes.org/advocacy

To find out how you can get involved with the programs in your community: Call 1-800-342-2383. See below for program Web addresses.

- *American Diabetes Month:* Educational activities aimed at those diagnosed with diabetes—month of November. www.diabetes.org/ADM
- *American Diabetes Alert:* Annual public awareness campaign to find the undiagnosed—held the fourth Tuesday in March. www.diabetes.org/alert
- *The Diabetes Assistance & Resources Program (DAR):* diabetes awareness program targeted to the Latino community. www.diabetes.org/DAR
- *African American Program:* diabetes awareness program targeted to the African American community. www.diabetes.org/africanamerican
- *Awakening the Spirit: Pathways to Diabetes Prevention & Control:* diabetes awareness program targeted to the Native American community. www.diabetes.org/awakening

To find out about an important research project regarding type 2 diabetes: www.diabetes.org/ada/research.asp

To obtain information on making a planned gift or charitable bequest: Call 1-888-700-7029. www.diabetes.org/ada/plan.asp

To make a donation or memorial contribution: Call 1-800-342-2383. www.diabetes.org/ada/cont.asp